Nuclear Medicine Hot Lab for Technologists

Nuclear Medicine Hot Lab for Technologists

Khalid Jassim

NM Techs™

Educational Recourses for Nuclear Medicine Technologists

DEDICATION

This work is a dedication to The Lady of Heaven.

ladyofheaven.com

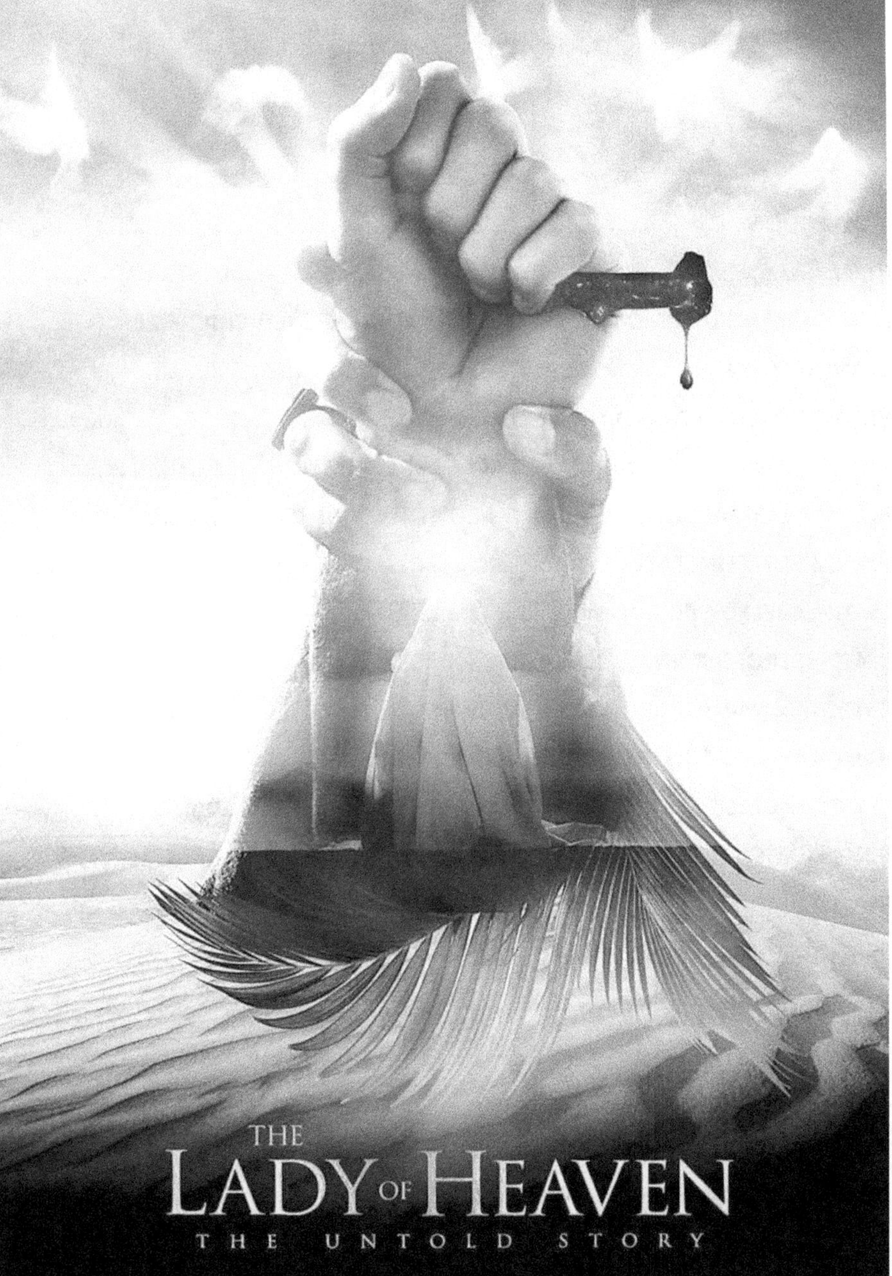

THE
LADY OF HEAVEN
THE UNTOLD STORY

CONTENTS

Introduction

"Nuclear Medicine Hot Lab for Technologist" is designed to be a valuable companion for nuclear medicine technologist and students in the field. Nuclear Medicine is a dynamic and essential branch of medical imaging, and this comprehensive guide is intended to facilitate within the hot lab, equipping you with the knowledge and skills necessary to excel in your role.

Throughout this handbook, you will find a wealth of information and practical insights, divided into three main sections. In the first part, we will explore label various pharmaceuticals with Technetium-99mTc, covering kits like MIBI, Tetrofosmin, MAA, Colloids, DMSA, DTPA, MAG-3 and others.

The second part of this handbook will explore haematology and common non imaging procedures in nuclear medicine. From the Carbon-14 Urea Breath Test to determining glomerular filtration rate using blood samples and even red and white blood cells labelling. We provide you with a comprehensive understanding of these techniques

The appendix offers a variety of common equations with examples, which simplify calculation of the activity and volume for the kits and patient dosage. Additionally, you will find essential guidelines on pharmacy radiation protection, best practices and waste management procedures, which are important for ensuring safety and efficiency in your work.

Whether you are a student starting your nuclear medicine journey or an experienced technologist seeking to refresh your knowledge and seeking to enhance your skills, this handbook aims to aid you on your pursuit.

Part 1

Radiopharmaceuticals Preparation in Nuclear Medicine

1 Introduction

In this part we will explore Technetium 99mTc elution from 99Mo/99mTc generator, quality control, and labeling 99mTc with different pharmaceuticals.

2 99Mo/99mTc Generator

99Mo/99mTc Generator

- In A 99Mo/99mTc generators the radioactive daughter (99m-Tc) can be separated by a simple chemical process, by liquid elution.
- 99Mo decays to its daughter radionuclide 99mTc as pertechnetate 99mTcO4.
- A 99Mo/99mTc generators consists of an alumina-filled column onto which 99Mo is absorbed.
- Generator elution is done by removing 99mTcO4 from the columns by drawing over saline from the column.
- The generator column and the whole system are well shielded with lead.
- The 99 Mo parent radionuclide decays, producing:
    - Metastable 99mTc with 87.5%intensity, which decays to 99Tc with a half-life of 6.02 h and emission of 140.5 Kev gamma radiations.
    - 99Tc with 12.5% intensity, which has a half-life of 212000 years to stable to ruthenium-99

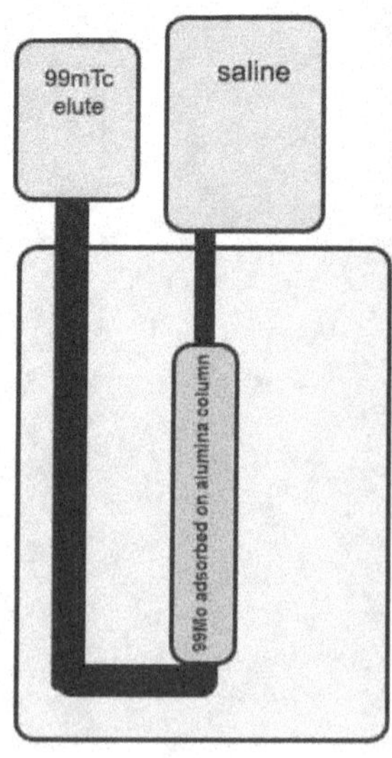

99Mo/99mTc generator

- The elute is a clear, colorless, isotonic solution of VII pertechnetate.
- Generators should be eluted regularly and completely to reduce the formation of the long lived 99Tc.

Generator Elute Quality control:

Radionuclide Purity:

- Mo is the most important impurity.
- The limit of contamination with Mo is 0.1% of the total elute activity.

Radiochemical Purity:

- Technetium may exist in seven oxidation states.
- In the 99mTc elute, the chemical species is 99mTc (VII) - pertechnetate.
- Not less than 95% of the radioactivity is identified as sodium pertechnetate [99mTc] by paper chromatography.
- Ascending thin-layer chromatography on silica gel glass fiber sheets is used for radiochemical purity analysis.
- Acetone is recommended as solvent.
- Sodium pertechnetate [99mTc] migrates with the solvent front (RF 1.0).
- Reduced, hydrolyzed activity is analyzed in saline (RF = 0).

Chemical Purity:

- Aluminum cations are formed during absorption of MO.
- A modified quinalizarin-based spot test is used for colorimetric evaluation of elutes against a known standard dilution.

PH of Elute:

- PH range should be between 4.0 and 8.0.

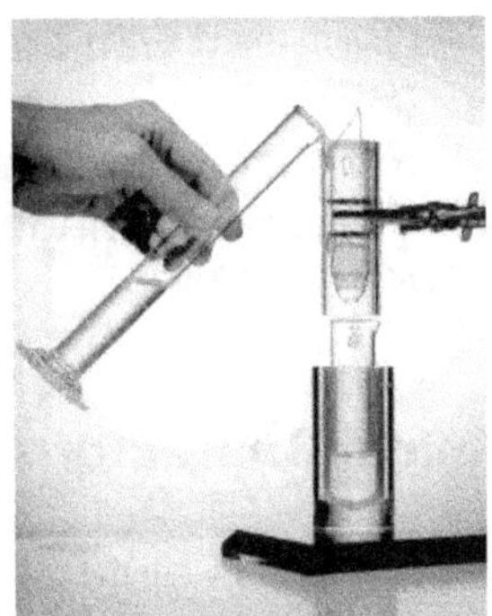

First 99Mo/99mTc generator 1958

3 Technetium 99m Tc Pharmaceuticals Preparation

Technetium-99m is widely used in radiopharmaceutical preparations due to its excellent physical and chemical properties.

physical Characteristics

- 99mTc decays with a half-life of 6 h and emission of 140.5-keV gamma radiation.
- Can used with the single-photon emission computed tomography (SPECT).
- Produce high-contrast images.
- The energy window of the gamma camera is optimized to 140.5 keV (110-220 keV).

Chemical Characteristics

- 99mTc is eluted from the generator as a pertechnetate anion.
- Technetium must be reduced to a lower state in order to be chemically reactive for labeling.
- Most 99m Tc pharmaceuticals comprise complexes of 99mTc at various oxidation states (I-V).

- The availability of commercial cold kits containing the chemical ingredients as a lyophilized formulation ready for labeling with 99mTc-pertechnetate.

Kit Preparations

- The preparation of any 99mTc pharmaceutical is performed by using a commercial cold kit and adding the required 99mTc activity in a certain volume of 99mTc elutes (pertechnetate).
- Cold kits offer convenience and ease of preparation for ad hoc labeling.
- The labeling procedure is termed as "reconstitution of the kit".

Radiolabeling

- Radiolabeling: is a process by which a new chemical compound (a 99mTc pharmaceutical) is formed involving chemical reactions.
- Labeling by a closed procedure: is a procedure where a sterile radiopharmaceutical is prepared by the addition of sterile ingredients to a pre sterilized closed container via a system closed to the atmosphere.
- 99mTc elute is added to the sterile vial (kit) with a syringe.
- An excess of pressure in the vial is avoided by withdrawing an equal volume of gas with the same syringe.
- A breather needle should not be used because oxygen may affect the stability of the radiopharmaceutical, and may cause microbial contamination.
- The instructions given by the manufacturer of the kit should be strictly followed.
- The labeled product is a sterile, pyrogenic free solution suitable for intravenous injection.
- Any abnormality observed by visual inspection of the injection solution is a cause to reject the preparation.
- 99mTc radiopharmaceuticals have a short shelf-life (generally 6 h); they are used right after preparation.

Cold Kits

- Cold kits are prepacked sets of sterile ingredients designed for the preparation of a specific radiopharmaceutical.
- Kits are fully tested and guaranteed by the producer.
- A kit contains the active ingredient, a reducing agent, and may contain authorized excipients and additives, such as antimicrobial agents, antioxidants, buffer, a nitrogen atmosphere, etc.
- The active ingredient: is the compound to be labeled with the radionuclide.
- The reducing agent: is responsible for the reduction of pertechnetate to a lower valency state. Without reduction, there is no labeling reaction.
- Freeze-drying was applied to kit production to ensure the stability of kits.
- Exact filling of the sterilized Kits vials is performed automatically by a sterile dispensing/stoppering device, whereby a certain volume (1 ml) of the kit formulation is delivered and subjected to lyophilization.
- When closing the vial, nitrogen gas is introduced through a sterile filter.
- Kit contents are stable for long periods.
- The shelf-life of kits is usually in excess of 1 year.
- It is important that kits are stored according to the specific conditions (temperature, humidity) indicated on the package, since radiolabeling depends on the integrity of the reducing agent.

99mTc elute pertechnetate

- The 99mTc elute used for radiolabeling must comply with the specifications stated in the pharmacopeia.
- The specific activity (activity/Tc carrier) and the activity concentration (activity/ml) should be known.
- Daily elution of the generator at an interval of 24 h will produce elutes with the best quality.
- The total 99mTc activity and the volume injected into the vial (kit) should comply with the recommendations by the manufacturer.
- Dilutions should be performed with isotonic saline.

Incubation:

- Incubation is an essential step to obtain the radiolabeled medicinal product, which is done after dissolving the lyophilisate in the added volume.
- In this phase, the chemical reactions take place, resulting in 99mTc labeling.
- If incubation is inadequate, the labeling reaction may not be completed, and the radiopharmaceutical may not be suitable for administration.
- Each kit requires specific incubation conditions, generally done at room temperature.
- In certain cases, the incubation must be performed in a boiling water bath.

Quality Control:

- Quality is directly related to the labeling yield, which is measured by the amount of unbound 99mTc activity.
- To assure safety and efficacy of a 99mTc radiopharmaceutical, the product should be tested regularly, before application to the patient.
- Radiochemical purity is analyzed by thin-layer chromatography.
- Poor quality of a radiopharmaceutical would affect the clinical information and cause unnecessary radiation exposure of a patient.

Dispensing:

- Is the compliance of a prescribed medicinal product with the required quality standards.
- For dispensing a prescribed amount of radioactivity, it is necessary to determine the total radioactivity and the radioactivity concentration of the radiopharmaceutical.
- A single dose may be withdrawn aseptically from the multi dose vial by using a suitable syringe.
- Each syringe must be measured in the dose calibrator to verify the prescribed amount of radioactivity for a patient.
- Syringes with individual doses of the radiopharmaceutical may be prepared in advance.

- The correct identification of each syringe is mandatory, stating on the label: Identification of patient (name and/or number) Name of the radiopharmaceutical Amount of radioactivity and time of preparation.

4 99m Tc Pharmaceuticals Quality Control Methods

Radiochemical Purity using Thin-Layer Chromatography (TLC):

- In this method a mobile phase (solvent) moves along a layer of adsorbent (stationary phase) due to capillary forces.
- A radioactive sample spotted onto the adsorbent will migrate with different velocities, and thus, impurities are separated.
- The distance each component of a sample migrates is expressed as the RF value.
- The Rf is the relative migration of a component in relation to the solvent front (SF):
- RF= Distance from origin of the component / Distance of the SF
- The RF values range from 0-1.
- If a component migrates with the SF, the Rf is 1.
- If a component remains at the point of application (origin), the Rf is O.
- The Rf value of a pure chemical compound is specific and reproducible.

The main impurities in 99mTc pharmaceutical preparations are:

1-free pertechnetate (99mTcO-4)
2-reduced, hydrolyzed technetium (colloidal 99mTc).

- These two Tc species may be separated from Tc pharmaceuticals by TLC procedures.
- The migration properties of free pertechnetate may be influenced by the choice of different mobile and stationary phases.

stationary phase:

- Instant TLC (ITLC) is the most used stationary phases in nuclear medicine.
- ITLC plates are made of fiberglass sheets, and an adsorbent, usually silica gel (SG).
- To separate and quantify two (or more) impurities, two (or more) analytical systems are used.
- Attention must be paid when ITLC strips are marked to indicate the spotting area or SF, since the material is fragile and easily damaged, which may affect results.

- To quantify free Tc-pertechnetate:
  - an organic solvent (MEK) or Acetone is used for separation
  - colloidal forms and the Tc complex remain at the origin
  - Free pertechnetate migrates with the SF.
- To quantify colloidal 99mTc:
  - saline is used for separation
  - free pertechnetate and the 99mTc complex migrate with the SF
  - reduced, hydrolyzed 99mTc remains at the start

Mobile phase:

- The saline/MEK system is applied for the analysis of most radiopharmaceuticals that contain free pertechnetate and/or colloidal Tc.

- Acetone has been replaced by MEK because artificially high values of pertechnetate have been obtained, caused by its higher water content.

Spotting the sample:

- The sample size has a considerable effect on the separation characteristics of a certain system.
- So, the sample diameter on the plate should be kept as small as possible (< 3 mm).
- Inefficient separations and artificial results are caused by too-large spots.
- To apply a sample onto the plate a micro pipets or capillaries for single use is used. The volume is typically 5 µl.
- To reduce handling, the sample is withdrawn using a 1 ml syringe with a fine needle (>25 gauge) and is spotted directly onto the plate using a single drop with volume 6 µl.
- If the syringe is held in the horizontal position, the volume might double.

Procedure for the determination of radiochemical purity by ITLC or paper chromatography:

- Fill a beaker with the solvent (about 10 ml, solvent 3-5mm high); close the beaker with a tight lid or para film.
- Prepare the strip.
- Mark the solvent front with a color pen and the Start with a pencil.
- Take a small sample of the preparation ready for injection 100 µl).
- Apply the sample with a thin needle onto the strip; the drop must not dry.
- Immediately put the strip into the beaker, the spot must remain above the solvent
- When the solvent has reached the front, take the strip out and let it dry.
- Quantify the regional distribution of radioactivity on the strip.

Radioactivity measurement:

- to calculate the radiochemical purity of a radiopharmaceutical percentage:

- Radiochemical purity (dpm)= (Radiopharmaceutical / Total recovered activity (dpm)) x100
- The strip is Cut into two segments (one corresponding to the main compound and the Other to the impurity) and measured in the ionization chamber.

5 99mTc-Pertechnetate

Chemical name

- Sodium pertechnetate
- Sodium pertechnetate 99mTc injection
- Technetium Tc 99m
- 99mTc (VII)-Na-pertechnetate

Physical characteristics

- Gamma energy=140.5 kev
  T1/2 = 6.02 hour

Preparation

- Sodium pertechnetate 99mTc is eluted from an approved 99M0/99mTc generator with Sterile, isotonic saline.
- Sodium pertechnetate 99mTc is a clear, colorless solution for intravenous injection.
- The pH value is 4.0-8.0.

Clinical Applications

99mTc(VII)-pertechnetate is used after intravenous injection in patients (70 kg) for:

- Thyroid scintigraphy: 75 MBq
- Salivary gland scintigraphy: 40 MBq
- Imaging of gastric mucosa (Meckel's diverticulum): 185 MBq
- Brain scintigraphy: 550 MBq, after blocking thyroid and choroid plexus to avoid nonspecific uptake of 99mTc pertechnetate
- Lacrimal duct scintigraphy: 2-4MBq instilled into each eye
- In vivo labeling of RBC: 740 MBq, after pretreatment with a stannous agent Dose.
    - Regional blood pool imaging
    - First-pass cardiac radionuclide angiography (ejection fraction, wall motion)
    - Detection of occult gastrointestinal bleeding

Quality Control

Radiochemical Purity

- More than 95% of 99mTc activity must be present as pertechnetate anion.

Thin-layer chromatography

- Solvent Acetone
- Chromatography Strip: Red
- free pertechnetate (99mTcO4), Rf= 0.9-1
- reduced, hydrolyzed technetium (colloidal 99mTc), Rf= 0-0.1
- 99mTc-pertechnetate, Rf= 0-0.1
- Radiochemical Impurity % = (free 99mTc Radioactivity / Total Radioactivity) x 100
- Radiochemical Purity % = 100 - (free 99mTc)
- e.g.
    - % free Tc = (1.2/ (1.2 + 99)) x 100 = 1.19 %
    - Radiochemical Purity % = 100 % - (1.19) % = 98.81%
    - Or Radiochemical Purity % = (99/ (1.2 + 99)) x 100 = 98.8 %

Radionuclide Purity (99Mo impurity).

- Generators are eluted after shipment, before administration of elutes to patients because
- The primary elute contains the highest concentration of chemical impurities and of Carrier 99Tc (decay product).
- parent 99M0 is highest in the first elute.

- a sample of the fresh elute (37 MBq) used to Determine 99MO impurity.

Pharmacokinetic Data

- Pertechnetate is actively transported into the thyroid in a manner similar to iodide by active transport
- it is not metabolized and is released from the thyroid unchanged.
- Uptake in the thyroid is between 1.5 and 2% Of the injected activity within 20 min
- iodinated contrast agents or iodine-containing medication would interfere with thyroid imaging.
- 99mTc pertechnetate is concentrating in the thyroid gland, salivary glands, gastric mucosa, choroid plexus, and mammary tissue.
- elimination of radioactivity; 50-60% are cleared with a half-time of 15 min;
- the remainder is eliminated more slowly, With half-times of approximately 3 h.
- After oral administration, the highest value of 99mTc activity in blood was reached within 30 min.
- Pertechnetate is excreted by the kidneys,
- Other pathways (saliva, gastric juice, milk, sweat, Lactating women secrete 10% of pertechnetate in milk.
- Pertechnetate crosses the placental barrier.
- pertechnetate is excreted in the feces.
- A total of 60% of the administered radioactivity is recovered in urine and feces in 72 h
- approximately 40% is retained in the body, mainly in the digestive tract.
- The whole-body biological half-time is estimated to be 53 h.
- 99mTc pertechnetate is excreted unchanged
- When thyroidal uptake of 99mTc-pertechnetate should be avoided, pretreatment with an oral dose of potassium perchlorate is used to inhibit uptake.

6 99mTc-Labeled MIBI

Chemical name

- 2-Methoxy-isobutyl-isonitrile (MIBI)
- Tc(I)-Hexakis(2-methoxy-isobutyl-isonitrile) tetrafluroroborate.
- Technetium Tc 99m sestamibi
- 99mTc-MIBI

Preparation

- Labeling is done by adding 99mTc-pertechnetate (up to 300 mCi) to the reaction vial.
- Volume added to the vial (1-3 ml)
- The vial should be heated in a boiling water bath for 10 min, upright position.
- Then it should be cooled for 10 min, upright position.
- 99mTc-sestamibi is a clear, colorless solution for intravenous injection.
- the pH value is 5.3-5.9.

Clinical Applications

99mTc-MIBI is used after intravenous injection for:
- Myocardial perfusion Studies, (7-27 mci).
- Breast imaging, (15-25 mCi).
- Parathyroid imaging, (13,5-18.9 mCi).

Quality Control

Radiochemical Purity:

- should be not less than 94% Of the total radioactivity.

Thin-layer chromatography

- Solvent ethyl acetate
- Chromatography Strip: Pink
- free pertechnetate (99mTcO4), Rf= 0-0.1
- reduced, hydrolyzed technetium (colloidal 99mTc), Rf= 0-0.1
- 99mTc-MIBI, Rf= 0.5-0.8
- Radiochemical Impurity % = (free 99mTc Radioactivity / Total Radioactivity) x 100
- Radiochemical Purity % = 100 - (free 99mTc)
- e.g.
  - % free Tc = (1.2/ (1.2 + 99)) x 100 = 1.19 %
  - Radiochemical Purity % = 100 % - (1.19) % = 98.81%
  - Or Radiochemical Purity % = (99/ (1.2 + 99)) x 100 = 98.8 %

Storage and Stability

- Storage: Kits and 99mTc-MIBI injection solution should be stored at 15-25 C.
- Stability: 99mTc-MIBI injection solution should be used within 10 h after labeling.

Pharmacokinetic Data

- 99mTc-MIBI accumulates in the viable myocardial tissue proportional to blood flow.
- The major metabolic pathway for clearance is the hepatobiliary tract.
- The elimination during 3 h from the liver is 76%; from the spleen, 67%; and from the lung, 49%.
- Malignant breast lesions show the highest uptake of 99mTc-MIBI.

7 99mTc-Tetrofosmin

Chemical name

- 1,2-bis(bis(2-ethoxyethyl)-phosphino)-ethane
- Tetrofosmin
- 99mTc-tetrofosmin
- Tc(V) dioxo diphosphine complex

Preparation

- Labeling is done by adding 99mTc-pertechnetate (30-240 mCi) to the reaction vial.
- Volume added to the vial (4-10 ml)
  The incubation should be at room temperature
- 99mTc-tetrofosmin is a clear, colorless solution for intravenous injection.
- the pH value is 7.5-9.

Clinical Applications

99mTc-tetrofosmin is used after intravenous injection for:
- myocardial perfusion studies (5-27 mci)

Quality Control

Radiochemical Purity:

- should be not less than 90% Of the total radioactivity.

Thin-layer chromatography

- Solvent ethyl acetate
- Chromatography Strip: Dark Green
- pertechnetate (99mTcO4), Rf= 0.1-0.9
- reduced, hydrolyzed technetium (colloidal 99mTc), Rf= 0-0.1
- 99mTc-tetrofosmin, Rf= 0.4-0.7
- Radiochemical Impurity % = (free 99mTc Radioactivity / Total Radioactivity) x 100
- Radiochemical Purity % = 100 - (free 99mTc)
- e.g.
  - % free Tc = (1.2/ (1.2 + 99)) x 100 = 1.19 %
  - Radiochemical Purity % = 100 % - (1.19) % = 98.81%
  - Or Radiochemical Purity % = (99/ (1.2 + 99)) x 100 = 98.8 %

Storage and Stability

- Storage: Kits and 99mTc-tetrofosmin injection solution should be stored at 2-8 C.
- Stability: 99mTc-tetrofosmin injection solution should be used within 8 h after labeling.

Pharmacokinetic Data

- 99mTc-tetrofosmin accumulates in the viable myocardial tissue proportional to blood flow.
- The major metabolic pathway for clearance is the hepatobiliary tract.

8 99mTc-Albumin Macroaggregates (MAA)

Chemical name

- human serum albumin (MAA)
- Technetium 99m Macrosalb
- 99mTc-MAA

Preparation

- Labeling is carried Out by adding aseptically sterile 99m Tc-pertechnetate to the vial with an activity (2.5-100 mCi).
- Volume added to the vial (2.5-10 ml)
- The lyophilized material Will dissolve by agitating the reaction vial The incubation should be 15 min, With occasional agitation
- albumin (MAA) is a pale-white suspension ready for intravenous injection.
- The pH of the suspension is 3.5-7.5.

Clinical Applications

Lung perfusion scintigraphy

- Pulmonary diseases (i.e., emphysema, chronic obstructive disease, pulmonary hypertension, fibrosis, acute arterial obstruction)

- The mechanism of lung retention of particles like MAA is capillary blockade.

Radio nuclide venography

- for the evaluation of deep vein thrombosis
- a special technique is used for injection into veins on the dorsum of each foot.

Time of Examination

- Lung perfusion scintigraphy. immediately after intravenous injection
- Scintigraphy of the lower extremities: shortly after bilateral intravenous injection

Recommended Activities:

- Lung scintigraphy (adults): 37-185 MBq (1-5 mCi)
- Scintigraphy of the lower extremities: 130-150 MBq (3.5-4.0 mCi).

Additional Information

- Macroaggregates of albumin must not be injected in patients with hypersensitivity to human albumin.
- the number of aggregated albumin particles administered for a lung scan should be reduced to the minimum for patients with:
    - severe pulmonary hypertension
    - right-to-left cardiac shunts.

Quality Control

Radiochemical Purity:

- Unbound radioactivity should be not less than 90% Of the total radioactivity.

Thin-layer chromatography

- Solvent Acetone
- Chromatography Strip: Red
- free pertechnetate (99mTcO4), Rf= 0.9-1
- reduced, hydrolyzed technetium (colloidal 99mTc), Rf= 0-0.1
- 99mTc-MAA, Rf= 0-0.1
- Radiochemical Impurity % = (free 99mTc Radioactivity / Total Radioactivity) x 100
- Radiochemical Purity % = 100 - (free 99mTc)

- e.g.
  - % free Tc = (1.2/ (1.2 + 99)) x 100 = 1.19 %
  - Radiochemical Purity % = 100 % - (1.19) % = 98.81%
  - Or Radiochemical Purity % = (99/ (1.2 + 99)) x 100 = 98.8 %

Storage and Stability

- Storage: Kits and 99mTc-MAA injection solution should be stored at 2-8 C.
- Stability: 99mTc-MAA injection solution should be used within 8 h after labeling.

Pharmacokinetic Data

- after intravenous injection 90% Of the technetium-99m MAA is extracted during the first pass and retained in lung capillaries and arterioles.
- Erosion and fragmentation reduce the Macroaggregates particle size, facilitating removal of Macroaggregates from the lung).
- Then the fragments are accumulated in the liver by phagocytosis
- The elimination of radioactivity from the lung is by half-times between 4 and 6 h.
- Accumulation in the liver is assumed to be 25%, With an uptake half-time of 6 h and an elimination half-time of 5 days.
- Excretion of released pertechnetate in the urine is reported as 40 ± in 24 h, and an additional 9.0 ± 3.8% up to 48 h.

9 99mTc-Labeled colloids (Micro colloids)

Chemical name

- Colloidal tin hydroxide
- Technetium tin colloid
- 99mTc-tin colloid

Preparation

- Labeling is done by adding a suitable volume of sterile 99mTc elute (2.7-27 mCi).
- Volume added to the vial (5 ml)
- The incubation should be at room temperature for 20 min.
- Mix before use.
- 99mTc-tin colloid is a sterile, pyrogenic free, opalescent solution suitable for intravenous injection.
- The pH is 4.0-6.0

Clinical Applications

- Liver and spleen scintigraphy: (4-5.4 mCi).
- Gastric emptying, solid meal: (1 mCi in egg)

Quality Control

Radiochemical Purity:

- should be not less than 95% Of the total radioactivity.

Thin-layer chromatography

- Solvent Acetone
- Chromatography Strip: Red
- free pertechnetate (99mTcO4), Rf= 0.9-1
- reduced, hydrolyzed technetium (colloidal 99mTc), Rf= 0-0.1
- 99mTc-Tin colloid, Rf= 0-0.1
- Radiochemical Impurity % = (free 99mTc Radioactivity / Total Radioactivity) x 100
- Radiochemical Purity % = 100 - (free 99mTc)
- e.g.
  - % free Tc = (1.2/ (1.2 + 99)) x 100 = 1.19 %
  - Radiochemical Purity % = 100 % - (1.19) % = 98.81%
  - Or Radiochemical Purity % = (99/ (1.2 + 99)) x 100 = 98.8 %

Storage and Stability

- Storage: Kits and 99mTc-Tin colloid injection solution should be stored at 2-8 C.
- Stability: 99mTc-Tin colloid injection solution should be used within 4 h after labeling.

Pharmacokinetic Data

- Intravenously injected colloids distribute by phagocytic function of the reticuloendothelial system (RES).
- colloidal particle size of 0.3-0.6 um:
  - 80-90% Of the radioactivity is seen in the liver,
  - 5-10% seen in the spleen
  - 5-9% in the bone
- Larger colloidal particles show increased splenic uptake
- smaller particles localize in the bone marrow
- Increased splenic uptake has been seen with decreased liver function
- The clearance half-time of colloid in patients Without liver or circulatory disorders was 2.57 - 2.64 min.
- 99mTc-tin colloid is eliminated from the macrophages and with half times of 71h for liver and 37 h for spleen.

10 99mTc-Labeled Nano Colloids

Chemical name

- 99mTc-Rhenium sulfide Nano colloid
- Tin(II) sulfide Nano colloid
- 99mTcsulfide Nano colloid
- 99mTc- Nano colloid

Preparation

- Labeling is done by adding a suitable volume of sterile 99mTc elute (5-150 mCi).
- Volume added to the vial (1-5 ml)
- The incubation should be at room temperature for 5-10 min.
- Mix before use.
- 99mTc-Nano colloid is a sterile, pyrogenic free, suitable for intravenous injection.

Clinical Applications

- Lymphoscintigraphy: Imaging 15 min after subcutaneous (interstitial) injection up to 1 h

- Visualization of lymph nodes between 2 and 6 h after injection, Recommended Activities (0.5-2.97 mCi per injection site, 0.2-0.3 per injection)
- Sentinel lymph node (SLN) scintigraphy: Imaging 5-10 min after Subdermal or peritumoral injection up to 6 h, Recommended Activities 50-80 MBq (1.3-2.2 mCi)
- Oral application:
  - Gastroesophageal scintigraphy, Recommended Activities 20-40MBq (0.5-1 mCi)
  - Esophageal motility disorders
  - Gastro-duodenal motor activity

Quality Control

Radiochemical Purity:

- should be not less than 95% Of the total radioactivity.

Thin-layer chromatography

- Solvent Acetone
- Chromatography Strip: Red
- free pertechnetate (99mTcO4), Rf= 0.9-1
- reduced, hydrolyzed technetium (colloidal 99mTc), Rf= 0-0.1
- 99mTc-Nano colloid, Rf= 0-0.1
- Radiochemical Impurity % = (free 99mTc Radioactivity / Total Radioactivity) x 100
- Radiochemical Purity % = 100 - (free 99mTc)
- e.g.
  - % free Tc = (1.2/ (1.2 + 99)) x 100 = 1.19
  - Radiochemical Purity % = 100 % - (1.19) % = 98.81%
  - Or Radiochemical Purity % = (99/ (1.2 + 99)) x 100 = 98.8 %

Storage and Stability

- Storage: Kits and 99mTc-Nano colloid injection solution should be stored at 2-8 C.
- Stability: 99mTc-Nano colloid injection solution should be used within 6 h after labeling.

Pharmacokinetic Data

- After injection Nano colloid is transported with the interstitial liquid through the lymphatic capillaries into the lymph ducts, and retained by the regional lymph nodes.
- Release of the colloid from the lymph nodes is slow and increasing with movement of the extremities.
- The maximal accumulation is reached 3 h after injection.
- Drainage from the interstitial injection site was between 1 and 35% in 24 h.

11 99mTc-DMSA

Chemical name

- Dimercaptosuccinic Acid (DMSA)
- Succimer
- 99mTc(III)-DMSA
- 99mTc(V)-DMSA

Preparation

- Labeling is done by adding a suitable volume of sterile 99mTc elutes, (up to 100 mCi).
- Volume added to the vial (1-6 ml)
- The incubation should be at room temperature for 10-15 min.
- 99mTc-DMSA is a sterile, pyrogenic free, clear, colorless solution suitable for intravenous injection.
- The pH is 2.3-3.5.

Clinical Applications

- 99mTc(III)-DMSA is used after intravenous injection for: Renal imaging, Examination time 1-3 h after injection up to 6 h, (1-3.2 mCi).
- 99mTc(V)-DMSA after intravenous injection for: Scintigraphy of medullary carcinoma of the thyroid (MCT), Examination time 2-4 h after injection, (10 mCi).

Additional Information

- For static imaging of the kidneys, the radiotracer is retained in the renal parenchyma by tubular fixation.
- Imaging should be delayed for 3 h after injection due to the slow transfer of activity from blood to kidney,
- A marked increase in hepatic activity may result from poor labeling conditions or the patient may have other medical conditions.
- The patient should be adequately hydrated after injection and before 99mTc-DMSA scintigraphy.

Quality Control

Radiochemical Purity:

- Unbound radioactivity should be not less than 95% Of the total radioactivity.

Thin-layer chromatography

- Solvent Acetone
- Chromatography Strip: Yellow
- free pertechnetate (99mTcO4), Rf= 0.9-1
- reduced, hydrolyzed technetium (colloidal 99mTc), Rf= 0-0.1
- 99mTc-DMSA, Rf= 0-0.1
- Radiochemical Impurity % = (free 99mTc Radioactivity / Total Radioactivity) x 100
- Radiochemical Purity % = 100 - (free 99mTc)
- e.g.
  - % free Tc = (1.2/ (1.2 + 99)) x 100 = 1.19 %
  - Radiochemical Purity % = 100 % - (1.19) % = 98.81%
  - Or Radiochemical Purity % = (99/ (1.2 + 99)) x 100 = 98.8 %

Storage and Stability

- Storage: Kits and 99mTc-DMSA injection solution should be stored at 2-8 C.
- Stability: 99mTc(III)-DMSA injection solution should be used within 4-8 h after labeling.

Pharmacokinetic Data

- After intravenous injection, 99mTc-DMSA is taken up in the renal parenchyma, showing high cortical affinity.
- In normal patients, both kidneys are visualized 1h after intravenous injection.
- the maximum accumulation in the renal cortex is reached 3 h after injection.
- 99mTc-DMSA is exclusively excreted in the urine as unchanged molecule.
- 99mTc(V)-DMSA accumulation was seen in both bone and soft tissue metastases.

12 99mTc-HMPAO

Chemical name

- 4,8-diaza-3,6,6,9- tetramethyl- undecane- 2,10-dione-bisoxime (HMPAO)
- D, L-Hexamethylpropylene amine oxime (D, L-HMPAO)
- Exametazime
- Technetium 99mTc exametazime
- 99mTc-HMPAO

Preparation

- Labeling is done by adding 99mTc-pertechnetate (30 mCi) to the reaction vial.
- The incubation should be at room temperature for 5 min.
- 99mTc-HMPAO is a clear, colorless solution for intravenous injection.
- the pH value is 9-9.8.
- Stabilization of the 99mTc-HMPAO complex with methylene blue/phosphate buffer Will extend in vitro stability up to 6 after labeling, stabilizer should be added to the reaction vial within 2 minutes of preparation.
- Fresh elution less than 30 minutes should be used for stabilizing protocol.

Clinical Applications

99mTc-HMPAO is used after intravenous injection for:

- brain scintigraphy (10-20 mci)

Quality Control

Radiochemical Purity:

- Unbound radioactivity should be not less than 80% Of the total radioactivity.

Thin-layer chromatography

- Solvent Ethyl Acetate
- Chromatography Strip: Gold
- pertechnetate (99mTcO4), Rf= 0.1-0.9
- reduced, hydrolyzed technetium (colloidal 99mTc), Rf= 0-0.1
- 99mTc-HMPAO, Rf= 0.4-0.7
- Radiochemical Impurity % = (free 99mTc Radioactivity / Total Radioactivity) x 100
- Radiochemical Purity % = 100 - (free 99mTc)
- e.g.
  - % free Tc = (1.2/ (1.2 + 99)) x 100 = 1.19 %
  - Radiochemical Purity % = 100 % - (1.19) % = 98.81%
  - Or Radiochemical Purity % = (99/ (1.2 + 99)) x 100 = 98.8 %

Storage and Stability

- Storage: Kits and 99mTc-HMPAO injection solution should be stored at 15-25 C.
- Stability:
  - 99mTc-HMPAO stable injection solution should be used within 4-6 h after labeling.
  - 99mTc-HMPAO unstable injection solution should be used within 30 minute after labeling.

Pharmacokinetic Data

- The lipophilic 99mTc-HMPAO complex can cross the BBB.
- Then a secondary 99mTc-D, L-HMPAOcomplex is formed which cannot pass the BBB and is trapped inside the brain and in blood cells.
- The radioactivity pattern remains constant for 24 h. Elimination from the brain is very slow, after 24 h, > 70% Of the tracer is still in the brain.

13 99mTc-Diphoshonates

Chemical name

- 99mTc-DPD (Dicarboxypropane diphosphonate)
  - 3,3-diphosphono-1 ,2- propane-dicarboxy acid tetrasodium salt (DPD)
  - 1,2-dicarboxypropane diphosphonate
- 99mTc-HDP (Hydroxymethylene diphosphonate)
  - Hydroxymethylene diphosphonic acid, disodium salt (HMDP, HDP)
  - Technetium Tc 99m oxidronate
- 99mTc-MDP (Methylene diphosphonate)
  - Methylene diphosphonic acid disodium salt (MDP)
  - Methylene diphosphonate
  - Technetium Tc 99m medronate

Preparation

- Labeling is done by adding (up to 500 mCi) 99mTc-pertechnetate.
- Volume added to the vial (3-10 ml)
- The incubation should be at room temperature for 5-20 min.
- 99mTc-Diphoshonate is a sterile, pyrogenic free, opalescent solution suitable for intravenous injection.
- The pH is 3.5-7.5

Clinical Applications

99mTc-Diphoshonate is used after intravenous injection for:
- Skeletal imaging with 99m Tc-diphosphonate complexes, (8-20 mci).
- Radionuclide angiography with 99mTc-RBC, (15-20 mci

Quality Control

Radiochemical Purity:

- should be not less than 95% Of the total radioactivity.

Thin-layer chromatography

- System 1:
  - Solvent Acetone
  - Chromatography Strip: Red
  - free pertechnetate (99mTcO4), Rf= 0.9-1
  - reduced, hydrolyzed technetium (colloidal 99mTc), Rf= 0-0.1
  - 99mTc-Diphoshonate, Rf= 0-0.1
- System 2:
  - Distilled H20
  - Chromatography Strip: Black
  - free pertechnetate (99mTcO4), Rf= 0.9-1
  - reduced, hydrolyzed technetium (colloidal 99mTc), Rf= 0-0.1
  - 99mTc-Diphoshonate, Rf= 0.9-1
- Radiochemical Impurity (system1) % = (free 99mTc Radioactivity / Total Radioactivity) x 100
- Radiochemical Impurity (system2) % = (hydrolyzed technetium Radioactivity / Total Radioactivity) x 100
- Radiochemical Purity % = 100 - (free 99mTc (system1) + hydrolyzed technetium (system2))
- e.g.
  - % free Tc = (1.2/ (1.2 + 99)) x 100 = 1.19 %
  - % HR Tc = (1.3/ (1.3 + 99)) x 100 = 1.29 %
  - Radiochemical Purity % = 100 - (1.19+1.29) = 97.52%

Storage and Stability

- Storage: Kits and 99mTc-Diphoshonate injection solution should be stored at 2-8 C.
- Stability: 99mTc-Diphoshonate injection solution should be used within 6 h after labeling.

Pharmacokinetic Data

- after intravenous injection, 45-50% Of 99mTc-diphosphonates (MDP, HDP, DPD) accumulate in the skeleton, and the rest is excreted in the urine.
- Maximum bone accumulation occurs 1 h after injection and remains constant for 72 h.
- Delay should be taken at least after 2h.
- An increase bone uptake is shown in the osteogenic activity.

14 99mTc-DTPA

Chemical name

- Diethylenetriaminepentaacete (DTPA) as Calcium trisodium salt
- Pentetate
- 99mTc-DTPA

Preparation

- Labeling is done by adding a suitable volume of sterile 99mTc elutes, up to (300 mCi).
- Volume added to the vial (2-10 ml)
- The incubation should be at room temperature for 15-30 min.
- 99mTc-DTPA is a sterile, pyrogenic free, clear, colorless solution suitable for intravenous injection.
- The pH is 4.0-7.5

Clinical Applications

- 99mTc-DTPA is used after intravenous injection for:

- Renal studies, (1-10 mCi).
- Determination of the GFR, (1-10 mCi).
- Cerebral scintigraphy based on leaks in the blood-brain barrier (BBB), (8.1-13.5 mCi).
- Localization of inflammatory bowel disease, (5-10 mCi).
- Inhalation scintigraphy to measure regional lung ventilation, (nebulized activity 30 mCi, breathing time 3-5 minutes).

Quality Control

Radiochemical Purity:

- Unbound radioactivity should be not less than 95% Of the total radioactivity.

Thin-layer chromatography

- System 1:
    - Solvent Acetone
    - Chromatography Strip: Red
    - free pertechnetate (99mTcO4), Rf= 0.9-1
    - reduced, hydrolyzed technetium (colloidal 99mTc), Rf= 0-0.1
    - 99mTc-DTPA, Rf= 0-0.1
- System 2:
    - Distilled H20
    - Chromatography Strip: Black
    - free pertechnetate (99mTcO4), Rf= 0.9-1
    - reduced, hydrolyzed technetium (colloidal 99mTc), Rf= 0-0.1
    - 99mTc-DTPA, Rf= 0.9-1
    - Radiochemical Impurity (system1) % = (free 99mTc Radioactivity / Total Radioactivity) x 100
    - Radiochemical Impurity (system2) % = (hydrolyzed technetium Radioactivity / Total Radioactivity) x 100
    - Radiochemical Purity % = 100 - (free 99mTc (system1) + hydrolyzed technetium (system2))
    - e.g.
        - % free Tc = (1.2/ (1.2 + 99)) x 100 = 1.19 %
        - % HR Tc = (1.3/ (1.3 + 99)) x 100 = 1.29 %
        - Radiochemical Purity % = 100 - (1.19+1.29) = 97.52%

Storage and Stability

- Storage: Kits and 99mTc-DTPA injection solution should be stored at 2-8 C.
- Stability: 99mTc-DTPA injection solution should be used within 6-8 h after labeling.

Pharmacokinetic Data

- After intravenous injection, 99mTc-DTPA enters the extravascular space within 4 min
- DTPA is removed from the circulation exclusively by the kidneys
- 99mTc-DTPA cannot pass through the intact BBB, but in areas where structural defects permit diffusion.
- Inhalation of 99m TC-DTPA as an aerosol shows free diffusion of the particles
    - (diameter of 0.5 um) to the lung periphery and
    - alveolar retention, larger droplets (> I um)
- 99mTc-DTPA reaching the blood is excreted by the kidneys.

15 99mTc-MAG3

Chemical name

- Benzoylmercapto-acetytriglycine: Betiatide
- 99mTc (V) O-mercaptoacetyltriglycine
- 99mTc-MAG3

Preparation

- Labeling is done by adding a suitable volume of sterile 99mTc elutes, up to (80 mCi).
- Volume added to the vial (3-10 ml)
- The vial should be heated in a boiling water bath for 10 min, upright position.
- Then it should be cooled for 10 min, upright position.
- 99mTc-MAG3 is a sterile, pyrogenic free, clear or slightly opalescent solution suitable for intravenous injection.
- The pH is 5.0-7.5

Clinical Applications

- 99mTc-MAG3 is used after intravenous injection for Renal imaging.
- Recommended Activities (1-5 mCi) are used in adults (70 kg).
- Studies of renal blood flow or transport through the ureters generally require a larger dose than do studies of intra-renal transport.

Additional Information

- The patient should be adequately hydrated before the scan because Insufficient Hydration of the patient Will affect the renal excretion rate.
- ACE inhibitors such as captopril maybe used for the differential diagnosis of Reno-vascular hypertension.
- diuretics such as furosemide (Lasix) cause rapid washout of the radiotracer or demonstrate urinary tract obstruction.

Quality Control

Radiochemical Purity:

- Unbound radioactivity should be not less than 94% Of the total radioactivity.

Thin-layer chromatography

- System 1:
    - Solvent Acetone: Chloroform 2:1
    - Chromatography Strip: Lime
    - free pertechnetate (99mTcO4), Rf= 0.9-1
    - reduced, hydrolyzed technetium (colloidal 99mTc), Rf= 0-0.1
    - 99mTc-MAG3, Rf= 0-0.1
- System 2:
    - Saline
    - Chromatography Strip: silica gel
    - free pertechnetate (99mTcO4), Rf= 0.9-1
    - reduced, hydrolyzed technetium (colloidal 99mTc), Rf= 0-0.1
    - 99mTc-MAG3, Rf= 0.9-1
    - Radiochemical Impurity (system1) % = (free 99mTc Radioactivity / Total Radioactivity) x 100
    - Radiochemical Impurity (system2) % = (hydrolyzed technetium Radioactivity / Total Radioactivity) x 100
    - Radiochemical Purity % = 100 - (free 99mTc (system1) + hydrolyzed technetium (system2))
    - e.g.
        - % free Tc = (1.2/ (1.2 + 99)) x 100 = 1.19 %
        - % HR Tc = (1.3/ (1.3 + 99)) x 100 = 1.29 %
        - Radiochemical Purity % = 100 - (1.19+1.29) = 97.52%

Storage and Stability

- Storage: Kits and 99mTc-MAG3 injection solution should be stored at 2-8 C.
- Stability: 99mTc-MAG3 injection solution should be used within 8 h after labeling.

Pharmacokinetic Data

- After intravenous injection, 99mTc-MAG3 is rapidly distributed in the extracellular fluid and excreted entirely by the renal system.
- The maximum renal accumulation of radioactivity is observed at 3-4 min after intravenous injection.
- The elimination from plasma is described by two half-times, 3.2 and 16 minutes.

16 99mTc-IDA

Chemical name

- N-(2,4,6-trimehtyl-3-bromophenylcarbamoylmethyl)-iminodiacetic acid (Mebrofenin)
- Etifenin
- Lidofenin
- Disofenin
- 99mTc-IDA

Preparation

- Labeling is done by adding a suitable volume of sterile 99mTc elute, (10-40 mCi).
- Volume added to the vial (5 ml)
- Mix for 2 minute.
- The incubation should be at room temperature for 30 min.
- 99mTc-IDA is a sterile, pyrogenic free, clear, colorless solution suitable for intravenous injection.
- The pH is 4-7.5.

Clinical Applications

- 99mTc-IDA is used after intravenous injection for Hepatobiliary imaging.
- Recommended Activities (3-5 mCi).

Additional Information

- The patient should not eat 2-6 h prior to the hepatobiliary scintigraphy, because hepatocyte clearance of the radiotracer and parenchymal transit time is affected by the ingestion of food.
- The gallbladder cannot be seen in 65% Of cases within the first 60 min of injection, even if the cystic duct is patent.
- Gallbladder contractility can be provoked with a fatty meal or intravenous cholecystokinin or sincalide.
- Narcotic (opioid) analgesics (morphine, meperidine) and phenobarbital cause a marked increase in biliary tract pressure, so a dose of morphine sulfate is administered intravenously, When the gallbladder has not been visualized within 60 min.
- Morphine should not be given to patients with a history of drug abuse, an allergy to morphine, or with pancreatitis.
- Phenobarbital enhances the biliary conjugation and excretion of bilirubin and promotes the excretion of organic anions such as 99mTc-IDA that are not conjugated by the liver, so it is may be given at least 5 days prior to the imaging.

Quality Control

Radiochemical Purity:

- Unbound radioactivity should be not less than 95% Of the total radioactivity.

Thin-layer chromatography

- System 1:
    - 20%NaCl (saline)
    - Chromatography Strip: Orange
    - free pertechnetate (99mTcO4), Rf= 0.9-1

- reduced, hydrolyzed technetium (colloidal 99mTc), Rf= 0-0.1
- 99mTc-IDA, Rf= 0-0.1

- System 2:
  - Water
  - Chromatography Strip: Light Blue
  - free pertechnetate (99mTcO4), Rf= 0.9-1
  - reduced, hydrolyzed technetium (colloidal 99mTc), Rf= 0-0.1
  - 99mTc-IDA, Rf= 0.9-1
  - Radiochemical Impurity (system1) % = (free 99mTc Radioactivity / Total Radioactivity) x 100
  - Radiochemical Impurity (system2) % = (hydrolyzed technetium Radioactivity / Total Radioactivity) x 100
  - Radiochemical Purity % = 100 - (free 99mTc (system1) + hydrolyzed technetium (system2))
  - e.g.
    - % free Tc = (1.2/ (1.2 + 99)) x 100 = 1.19 %
    - % HR Tc = (1.3/ (1.3 + 99)) x 100 = 1.29 %
    - Radiochemical Purity % = 100 - (1.19+1.29) = 97.52%

Storage and Stability

- Storage: Kits and 99mTc-IDA injection solution should be stored at 2-8 C.
- Stability: 99mTc-IDA injection solution should be used within 5 h after labeling.

Pharmacokinetic Data

- Most of 99mTc-IDA injected dose are extracted by the hepatocytes and secreted into bile.
- In patients with normal hepatobiliary function, maximal liver uptake is measured at about 12 min.
- The gallbladder is well visualized 20 min post injection.
- Intestinal activity appears on the average at 15-30 min.
- The common bile duct may be visualized after 14 min.
- The upper limit of visualization of these structures is 1 h.

17 99mTc-Pyrophosphate (PYP)

Chemical name

- Sodium pyrophosphate, 10H2o (PYP) Tin(II) diphosphate
- Technetium 99mTc tin pyrophosphate
- Technetium 99mTc pyrophosphate
- 99mTc-PYP

Preparation

- The vial is reconstituted with sterile saline or with sterile sodium 99mTc-pertechnetate injection solution.
- Following reconstitution, the vial is agitated.
- (99mTc-PYP) solution is clear and free of particulate matter.
- the pH value is 5.0-7.0.
- Pretreatment of red blood cells (RBC) With PYP for in vivo labeling with 99mTc:
    - Stannous pyrophosphate cold kits are used for in vivo labeling of erythrocytes with 99mT pertechnetate.
    - In this case, the vial is reconstituted with (3-10 ml) saline or water.
    - The incubation should be 5 min at room temperature.
    - 3.0-4.0 mg of stannous pyrophosphate is injected intravenously
    After 30 min, (15-20 mCi) is injected intravenously, for in vivo labeling of pretreated erythrocytes

Clinical Applications

99mTc-PYP is used after intravenous injection for:
- Regional imaging of blood pools (deep vein visualization)
- Electrocardiogram cardiac radionuclide ventriculography (ejection fraction, wall motion) Detection of gastro intestinal hemorrhage, blood loss.
- Determination of RBC mass or blood volume.
- Spleen scintigraphy (heat treated labeled RBC).

Quality Control

Radiochemical Purity:

- should be not less than 90% Of the total radioactivity.

Thin-layer chromatography

- Solvent Acetone
- free pertechnetate (99mTcO4), Rf= 0.9-1
- reduced, hydrolyzed technetium (colloidal 99mTc), Rf= 0-0.1
- 99mTc-PYP, Rf= 0-0.1
- Radiochemical Impurity % = (free 99mTc Radioactivity / Total Radioactivity) x 100
- Radiochemical Purity % = 100 - (free 99mTc)
- e.g.
    - % free Tc = (1.2/ (1.2 + 99)) x 100 = 1.19 %
    - Radiochemical Purity % = 100 % - (1.19) % = 98.81%
      Or Radiochemical Purity % = (99/ (1.2 + 99)) x 100 =

Storage and Stability

- Storage: PYP kit solution should be stored at 2-8 C.
- Stability: 99mTc-PYP injection solution should be used within 4h after labeling.

Pharmacokinetic Data

- After intravenous injection, 99mTc-PYP accumulates in regions of active osteogenesis, and also in injured myocardium, mainly in necrotic tissue
- The average urinary excretion is 60% Of the administered dose in 24 h.
- Stannous pyrophosphate has an affinity for RBC. It binds to the B-chain of hemoglobin.

20 Non- 99mTc radiopharmaceuticals

Some other Non- 99mTc radiopharmaceuticals includes:

Radioiodine-Labeled Radiopharmaceuticals (I131 and I123)

- Iodine-131 (8.02 days' half-life) is used in the treatment of hyperthyroidism and thyroid cancer.
- I123 (13-hour half-life and160-keV γ-ray emission) is used for diagnostic purposes.
- Iodine-131- or Iodine-123-Labeled Sodium Iodide: is available as a capsule or solution and are used for diagnosis of thyroid disease

I123-Hippuran:

- is used to study renal function.

Iodine-123-isopropylamphetamine (Spectamine):

- is used for measuring brain function.

I123/131-Metaiodobenzylguanidine (MIBG)

- used to:
    - detect and treat tumors of neuroendocrine origin.
    - disorders of sympathetic innervation.

I123-ioflupane (DAT):

- is used for the differential diagnosis between essential tremor and degenerative parkinsonism.

Gallium-67 Citrate

- Ga-67 (3.26 days' half-life and (93.3, 184.8, 300.2, 393.5-keV γ-ray emission) is used in detection of soft tissue tumors and inflammatory diseases.

Thallium-201 Chloride

- Thallous-201 Chloride (3.038 days' half-life) and (60-80, 135, 167-keV γ-ray emission) is used for detection of myocardial infarction and/or ischemia.

Chromium-51-Labeled Red Cells

- Cr-51 Labeled RBC used to determine the red cell volume and red cell mean life.

Indium-111-Labeled DTPA

- Used for imaging cerebrospinal fluid dynamics (injected intrathecal).
- (T½ = 2.8 days) and (173, 247-keV γ-ray emission)

Indium-111-Oxine Labeled Platelets and Leukocytes

- These are used for thrombus and abscess detection, respectively.

Indium-111-Labeled DTPA Pentetreotide (OctreoScan)

- Used for the detection of somatosin receptor-containing tumors.

Radiolabeled Monoclonal Antibodies and Synthetic Peptides

- Used for diagnosis and therapy of cancer and its metastases.
- used for diagnosis by labeling antibodies with radionuclides such as 111In and 99mTc or for therapy with 131

Part 2

Haematology & Non Imaging Procedures in Nuclear Medicine

1 Introduction

Nuclear Medicine procedures are used for diagnosis of a variety of haematological disorders and help in the diagnosis of many diseases without the need for traditional imaging techniques. This section will provide a detailed step-by-step exploration of these essential procedures.

- Equipment required for nuclear haematology is very simple such as:
  - Well scintillation counters to measure radioactivity in blood samples.
  - Gamma camera is required when imaging is necessary.

Radionuclides and blood elements labelling

- Radionuclides used for Labelling of various blood elements are Cr-51, Tc-99m and In-111.

  - Tc-99m:
    - Half-life: 6 hours
    - Emission: 140 KeV
    - Suitable for imaging: YES
  - In-111:
    - Half-life: 67.9 days
    - Emission: 171,247 KeV
    - Suitable for imaging: YES
  - Cr-51:
    - Half-life: 27.7 days
    - Emission: 320 KeV
    - Suitable for imaging: No

- Radionuclides used in blood labelling should have the following characteristics:

(a) It should not alter the function or the life span of the cell.

(b) It should not be reutilized after destruction of the cell.

(c) It should be a gamma emitter with appropriate energy and a half life appropriate to the studied subject.

Erythrocyte (Red Blood Cells) labelling

- Most commonly used radionuclide for erythrocyte labelling: Cr-51, Tc-99m, P-32, H-3, C-14

Leucocyte (White Blood Cells) labelling

- Most commonly used radionuclide for Leucocyte labelling: Tc-99m, P-32, H-3

Albumin or plasma labelling

Thrombocyte (platelet) labelling

- Most commonly used radionuclide for Leucocyte labelling: Cr-51, P-32, S-35, In-111

Types of cell labelling

Cohort labelling (pulse labelling):

- Is performed on cell precursors. The labelled precursors will appear in the circulation as labelled young cells and will remain in circulation throughout the life-span of the cell. Radioactive iron, perhaps, is the only radionuclide that is used for this type of labelling, but it is rarely available.

Random labelling:

- The radionuclide labels all cells of different degrees of maturity in a blood sample. This method requires separation of unbound label from the labelled fraction, which is done by centrifugation.

Tc-99m Red Blood Cells labeling Procedure:

Tinning:

- adding stannous ion (reduction agent) to RBCs, and Sn2+ diffuse into RBCs.
- stannous ion usually in a complex with Pyrophosphate or medronate, to prevent stannous ion removal from the blood by hydrolysis and precipitation.
- Stannous ion-PYP kit patient dose calculation mg/kg = Patient weight X 0.02
- Stannous ion-PYP kit prepared by adding 2-4 ml saline to it, then injected to the patient.

Labeling:

- Tc-99m added to tinned RBCs usually after 20-30 minute of Sn-PYP injection.
- Sn2+ reduce TC-99m from 7 to 4 oxidation state, which allow Tc-99m to bind to the Beta-globin chains of Hemoglobin.

Tc-99m Red Blood Cells labeling Methods:

In vivo / In vivo:

- Sn-PYP injected to the patient.
- After 20-30-minute Tc-99m injected to the patient and wait for 10 minutes.
- Labeling Efficiency 80-85%.

In vivo / In vitro (in vivitro):

- Sn-PYP injected to the patient.
- After 30 minute 5-10 ml blood drown from the patient, with a syringe that contain ACD-A.
- Tc-99m added to Blood syringe.
- Dose reinjected to the patient after at least 10 minutes.
- Labeling Efficiency 92%.

Modified in vivo / in vitro:

- Sn-PYP injected to the patient.
- After 20 minute 5-10 ml blood drown from the patient, with a syringe that contain ACD-A.
- Blood is centrifuged 5miutes-3000 RPM.
- Supernatant removed.
- Tc-99m added to Blood.
- Dose reinjected to the patient after at least 10 minutes.
- Labeling Efficiency 98%.

In vitro / in vitro:

- Blood drown from the patient, with a syringe that contain ACD-A.
- Blood is centrifuged 5miutes-3000 RPM.
- Supernatant removed.
- Sn-PYP added to Blood.
- After 20-minute Tc-99m added to Blood.
- Dose reinjected to the patient after at least 10 minutes.
- Labeling Efficiency 95%.

In vitro / in vitro (Ultra tag kit):

- Blood drown from the patient, with a syringe that contain ACD-A.
- Blood added to Ultra tag vial.
- After 5 minute Add syringe 1 & Add syringe 2 to the vial.
- Add Tc-99m added to the vial.
- Dose reinjected to the patient after at least 15 minutes.
- Labeling Efficiency 97%.

Calculate Labeling Efficiency:

- Draw 0.2 ml labeled RBC.
- Add 2 ml saline
- Centrifuge for 5 minute, at 3000 RPM.
- Remove supernatant and count.
- Count pellet.
- Labeling Efficiency % = (pellet activity/pellet activity+ supernatant activity)) x 100

2 Carbon-14 Urea Breath Test

Carbon-14 (C-14) urea breath test is used to detect the presence of Helicobacter pylori (H. pylori) in the stomach.

Patient preparation:

- The patient should fast 6 h before the study.
- The patients should brush teeth before the test.
- The patient should stop:
    - Antibiotics and bismuth compounds for 30 days
    - sucralfate and proton-pump inhibitors for 2 weeks before the test.
    - smoking overnight.

Procedure steps:

- Patient swallow 1 µCi C-14 urea capsule, with 20 ml water.
- After 3-minute patient drink 20 ml water.

Breath Collection:

- After 10 to 20 minute of capsule admin, the patient takes a deep breath and exhale in a Mylar balloon by straw.
- Close the balloon

Breath Analysis:

- Add 2.5 ml trapping solution (collection fluid-blue color) to a vial.
- Use the pump to transfer the air from the balloon to the vial until it become colorless.
- Add 10 ml scintillation fluid (cocktail) to the vial, and mix it.
- After 10 to 20-minute count using Liquid Scintillation Counter.
- Counting using the Liquid Scintillation Counter:
- Count standard and background samples,
- then calculate %Efficiency:

$$\%\text{Efficiency} = \frac{(Standard\ cpm - background\ cpm)}{20000\ Standard\ dpm} * 100$$

- Count patient sample using the Liquid Scintillation Counter
- Calculate patient sample:

$$\text{Dpm Sample} = \frac{(Sample\ cpm - background\ cpm)}{\%Efficiency}$$

Results:

- <50 dpm negative for H. pylori.
- 50-199 dpm indeterminate for H. pylori, the sample should be recounted in 1-2 h or the next day, to exclude falsely elevated counts due to chemiluminescence.
- ≥200 dpm is positive for H. pylori.

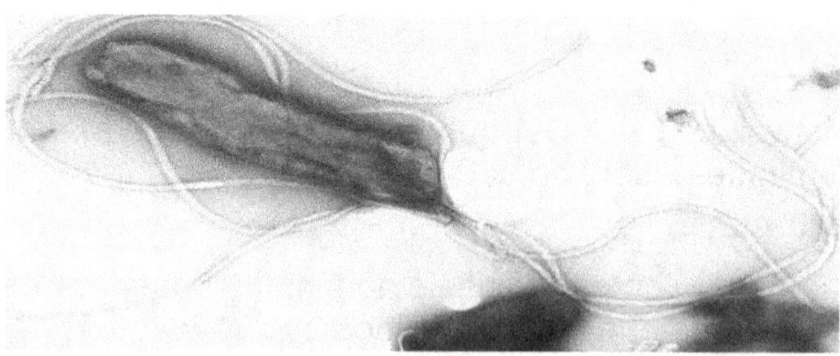

H. Pylori

3 Glomerular filtration Rate (GFR Blood Samples)

Glomerular filtration Rate or GFR is used to measure renal function. It can be camera based or blood based. Radiopharmaceuticals used include Tc-99m DTPA or Cr51-EDTA.

GFR measurement using Tc-99m DTPA & slope intercept method:

Patient Preparation:

- Hydrated at least 1000 ml water
- Stop caffeine
- Height and weight should be measured to determine BSA.

DTPA KIT PREPARE:

- ADD TC-99m (50-100) mCi to DTPA Vial
- MIX and INCUBATE (15 min)

DOSE DRAW:

- draw standard dose 1 mCi

- draw patient dose 10 mCi
- measure ALL the doses at the same time, better within 1min

EMPTY SYRINGE MEASURE:

- Measure empty patient dose with the cannula (remaining dose).

STANDARD PREPARTION:

- Add water to 1000 ml FLASK.
- Add the 1 mCi standard dose to the flask.

TUBES PREPARTION:

- Label 3 test tubes for standard 1, 2, 3.
- Label 3 test tubes for patient (2hour, 3 hours, 4 hour samples).
- Label 3 (2,5 ml filtered tubes) for patient (2hour, 3 hours, 4 hour samples).

BLOOD SAMPLES CENTRIFUGE:

- Draw 5-10 ml blood @ 2hr, 3hr, 4hr
- After receiving each patient sample, incubate for 30 minute
- Then centrifuge for 30 minute with 2 rpm.
- Then remove the plasma and add it to the 2,5 ml tube.
- Add the filter to the 2,5 ml tube and Then centrifuge for 20 minute with 2 rpm.
- Use 100 micro pipette to draw 100 micros from the filtered tube to the patient test tube.
- Repeat the steps for all the patient blood samples.
- Use 100 micro pipette to draw 100 micros from the 1000 ml flask to each of three standard test tubes.

Counting:

- Use multi-well counter to count the standard and patient test tubes.
- Blood based GFR is calculated using these readings.

Camera based GFR Imaging part:

- Full Dose syringe static image is taken for 30 sec
- Dynamic image for 21 minute for the kidneys is taken immediately after injection.
- Empty Dose syringe static image is taken for 30 sec
- Post void static image is taken for 2 minute
- Injection site static image is taken for 30 sec.
- Camera based GFR is calculated by processing the images using software.

4 White Blood Cells IN-111-oxine

Indications:

- osteomyelitis.
- Detection and localization of acute abscesses (e.g., liver, renal, intra-abdominal sepsis).
- fever of unknown origin [FUO]).
- inflammatory bowel disease.
- prosthesis rejection.
- pulmonary infections.

Procedure steps:

1. Draw 50ml blood from the patient slowly, in a syringe (at least 20 G) that contain 7 ml (ACD-A).
2. Flush the cannula with 10 ml saline and a drop of heparin.
3. Transfer the blood to two 25 ml falcon tubes
4. Add 7 ml (10% HES) Hydroxy-ethyl-starch to the two tubes and mix them.

5. Keep the two tubes for sedimentation for 30-45 minute, then tilt them 45°.
6. Use a Pasteur pipette to remove all the supernatant, then transfer it to a new falcon tube.
7. Centrifuge the new falcon tube for 5m minute, at 1000 RPM (150 g).
8. Remove the supernatant from the centrifuged blood and discard it.
9. Add 10 ml saline to the remaining pellet and mix, then centrifuge it for 5m minute, at 1000 RPM.
10. Remove the supernatant from the centrifuged blood and discard it.
11. Prepare IN-111-oxine (0.3- 0.5 mCi) patient dose, and add tris-buffer to it and mix it.
12. Add the dose to the falcon tube, and incubate it for 15 minute and mix it frequently.
13. Add 4 ml saline to the falcon tube, then centrifuge it for 5m minute, at 1000 RPM.
14. Remove supernatant and count it.
15. Count the pellet in the falcon tube.
16. QC 1: Calculate Labeling Efficiency, (should be > 75 %).
    Labeling Efficiency % = (pellet activity/pellet activity+ supernatant activity)) x 100
17. QC 2: Visual inspect for clots and clumps.
18. Add 4 ml saline to the falcon tube and mix it.
19. Draw all the patient Dose and inject immediately.
20. QC 3: Done after imaging: check early lung uptake and liver to spleen activity ratio.

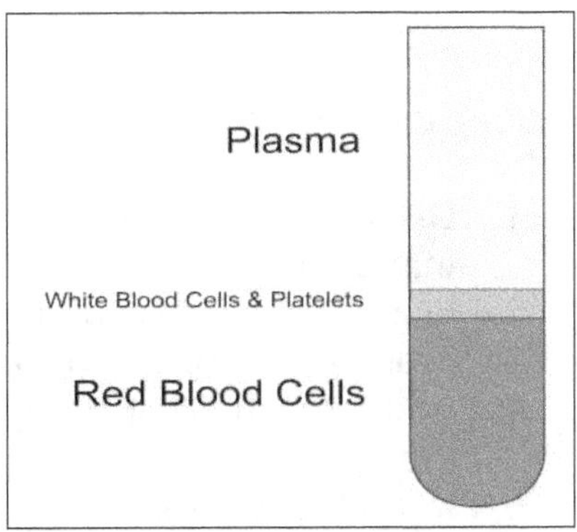

centrifuged blood

5 White Blood CellsTc-99m HMPAO

Indications:

- osteomyelitis.
- Detection and localization of acute abscesses (e.g., liver, renal, intra-abdominal sepsis).
- fever of unknown origin [FUO]).
- prosthesis rejection.
- pulmonary infections.

Procedure steps:

1. Draw 50ml blood from the patient slowly, in a syringe (at least 20 G) that contain 7 ml (ACD-A).
2. Flush the cannula with 10 ml saline and a drop of heparin.
3. Transfer the blood to two 25 ml falcon tubes
4. Add 7 ml (10% HES) Hydroxy-ethyl-starch to the two tubes and mix them.
5. Keep the two tubes for sedimentation for 30-45 minute, then tilt them 45°.

6. Use a Pasteur pipette to remove all the supernatant, then transfer it to a new falcon tube.
7. Centrifuge the new falcon tube for 5m minute, at 1000 RPM (150 g).
8. Remove the supernatant (plasma) from the centrifuged blood and discard it.
9. Add 10 ml saline to the remaining pellet and mix, then centrifuge it for 5m minute, at 1000 RPM.
10. Remove the supernatant from the centrifuged blood and discard it.
11. Prepare Tc-99m HMPAO, and draw patient dose.
12. Add the dose (5-10) mCi in 1 ml to the white blood cells falcon tube, and incubate it for 10 minute and mix it frequently.
13. Add 4 ml saline to the falcon tube, then centrifuge it for 5m minute, at 1000 RPM.
14. Remove supernatant and count it.
15. Count the pellet in the falcon tube.
16. QC 1: Calculate Labeling Efficiency, (should be > 75 %).
    Labeling Efficiency % = (pellet activity/pellet activity+ supernatant activity)) x 100
17. QC 2: Visual inspect for clots and clumps.
18. Add 5 ml saline to the falcon tube and mix it.
19. Draw all the patient Dose.
20. QC3: Done after imaging: check early lung uptake and liver to spleen activity ratio.

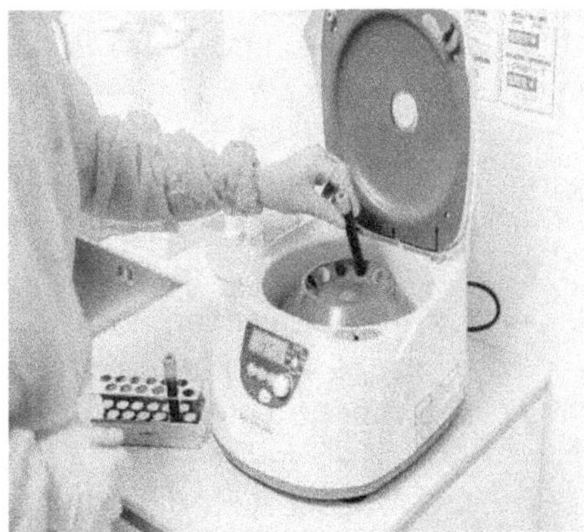

A centrifuge

6 Tc-99m Heat-Damaged Red Blood Cell

This study is done to evaluate the spleen and the accessory splenic tissue.

Procedure steps:

- Add 4ml saline to PYP vial and mix.
- Calculate PYP patient Dose = 0.02 x patient weight.
- Inject PYP to the patient.
- After 30-minute draw 6 ml blood from the patient, with a syringe that contain 1 ml (ACD-A).
- Transfer blood to Red Vacutainer Tube.
- Centrifuge for 5m minute, at 2500 RPM.
- Remove the plasma and discard it.
- Add saline (saline volume equal the discarded plasma).
- Add (1–6 mCi) Tc-99m to the Red Tube and mix it.
- Incubate the Red Tube for 35 minute in a 49.5 °C heated water bath.
- Calculate Labeling Efficiency, (should be 90-95 %).
  - Draw 1 ml blood.
  - Centrifuge for 5 minute, at 1300 RPM.

- o Remove supernatant and count.
- o Count pellet.
- o Labeling Efficiency % = (pellet activity/pellet activity+ supernatant activity)) x 100
- After calculating the patient dose (1-2 mCi), the heat damaged blood is reinjected to the patient.
- After 30 min to 1 h from injection imaging is done.
- static images or a SPECT or SPECT/CT on the spleen images is taken.

- Notes:
  - o If heating temperature is low, blood pool activity is high.
  - o If heating time is prolonged, liver uptake is high.

7 Red Blood Cells labelling Modified (In vivo-in vitro)

Indications:

- Gastrointestinal bleeding.
- Hepatic Hemangioma.

Procedure steps:

- Prepare PYP vail by adding 4 ml saline to it and mix it.
- Calculate PYP patient dose, then inject it.
    - PYP patient dose = 0.02 mg/kg x patient weight.
- After 30-minute draw 3-5 ml blood, with a syringe that contain 0.5 ml (ACD-A) and mix it.
- Prepare 25 mCi TC-99m dose and transfer it to Blood syringe (syringe to syringe transfer)
- Mix it and incubate for 15 minute
- Calculate Labeling Efficiency, (should be 92 %).
    - Draw 0.3 ml blood.
    - Add 2 ml saline
    - Centrifuge for 5 minute, at 3000 RPM.
    - Remove supernatant and count.

- o Count pellet.
  - o Labeling Efficiency % = (pellet activity/pellet activity+ supernatant activity)) x 100
- inject it to the patient.

Imaging Procedures for GI bleeding:

- Dynamic 60 minute.
- static images or a SPECT or SPECT/CT images is taken.

Imaging Procedures for Liver Hemangioma:

- Dynamic 3 minute.
- static images or a SPECT or SPECT/CT images is taken.

8 Red Blood Cells labelling Ultra-Tag (In vitro-in vitro)

Indications:

- Gastrointestinal bleeding.
- Hepatic Hemangioma.

Procedure steps:

- Draw 3 ml blood, with a syringe that contain 0.4 ml (ACD-A) and mix it.
- Transfer the blood to Ultra-Tag vial (reaction vial), and draw the same amount of air
- Mix it and incubate it for 5 minute
- Assemble Syringe 1 & 2 and keep syringe 1 away from light
- After 5-minute incubation:
- Add syringe 1 (Sodium hypochlorite) to Ultra-Tag vial, and draw the same amount of air and mix it.
- Add syringe 2 (Citric acid & dextrose solution) to Ultra-Tag vial, and draw the same amount of air and mix it.
- Add 25 mCi TC-99m to Ultra-Tag vial, and draw the same amount of air and mix it.

- Incubate it for 20 minute.
- Calculate Labeling Efficiency, (should more than 95 %).
    - Draw 0.3 ml blood.
    - Add 2 ml saline
    - Centrifuge for 5 minute, at 3000 RPM.
    - Remove supernatant and count.
    - Count pellet.
    - Labeling Efficiency % = (pellet activity/pellet activity+ supernatant activity)) x 100
- Draw patient dose.

Imaging Procedures for GI bleeding:

- Dynamic 60 minute.
- static images or a SPECT or SPECT/CT images is taken.

Imaging Procedures for Liver Hemangioma:

- Dynamic 3 minute.
- static images or a SPECT or SPECT/CT images is taken.

9 Red Cell Mass (RCM) and Plasma Volume (PV)

Measurements

Indication:

- polycythemia Vera.
- Anemia.
- trauma and burns.
- blood loss/replacement therapy.
- preoperative elderly patient.

Procedure:

A. RCM is measured using chromium-51.
B. PV is measured using I-125-HAS (Human Serum albumin).

Patient preparation:

- The patient should have had no transfusions or phlebotomy within the last 4 weeks.

- The patient has not had a radioisotope test in recent past.
- The patient should have a good breakfast before study.
- Height and weight should be measured.

RCM using chromium-51 Procedure steps:

- 10 ml blood is withdrawn into a heparinized syringe.
- Transfer blood to a sterile tube.
- Add Cr-51 (100 µCi) to the tube.
- Incubate for 20-30 minute.
- Centrifuge for 5 minute, 2500 RPM.
- Remove the supernatant & add the same amount of saline & mix.
- Withdraw 50 µCi Cr-51 labelled blood.
- Reinject to the patient.
- Collect 10 ml blood at 30, 60 and 90-minute post injection from a different vein.

Standard preparation:

- Draw 1 ml Cr-51 labelled blood from the prepared tube.
- Add 49 ml water to a measurement cylinder.
- Add the 1 ml Cr-51 labelled blood to the measurement cylinder.
- Volume 50 ml, Dilution Factor 50.

Measuring blood Hematocrit (HCT):

Hematocrit (HCT)= RED CELL VOLUME / TOTAL BLOOD VOLUME
PLASMACRIT = 1 - HCT

- Use a micro hematocrit centrifuge and a micro hematocrit reader to measure HCT as decimal.
- Measure HCT for each 30, 60 and 90-minute blood samples
- Total Blood Volume (TBV) = RCM / (0.9xHCT)

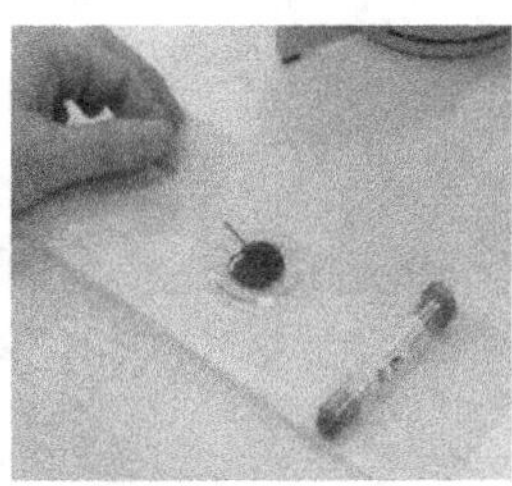

micro hematocrit tube

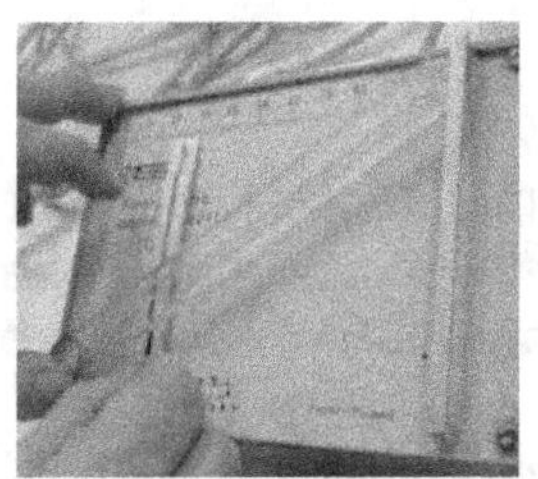

micro hematocrit reader

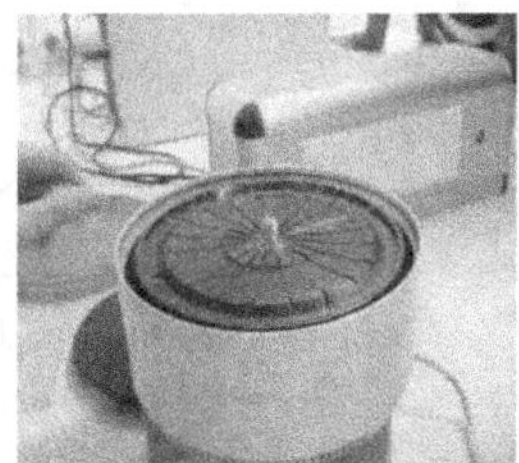

micro hematocrit centrifuge

Red Cells Volume:

- Prepare 10 polystyrene tubes:
  - Tube 1: pipette 1 ml water (for background)
  - Tube 2: 1 ml from the standard 50 ml measurement cylinder.
  - Tube 3: 1 ml from the standard 50 ml measurement cylinder
  - Tube 4: 1 ml 30-minute whole blood sample.
  - Tube 5: 1 ml 60-minute whole blood sample.
  - Tube 6: 1 ml 90-minute whole blood sample.

- Centrifuge the blood sample:
  - Tube 7: 1 ml standard plasma
  - Tube 8: 1 ml 30-minute plasma
  - Tube 9: 1 ml 60-minute plasma
  - Tube 10: 1 ml 90-minute plasma
- Count the 10 tubes in a well counter
- spectrometer center 320 KeV.
- photo peak of Cr-51.
- Count Time 300 seconds.

Calculation:

- Anticipated RCM for Male = ((8.2 x height) + (17.3 x weight)) - 693 ± 504
- Anticipated RCM for Female = ((16.4 x height) + (5.7 x weight)) - 1649 ± 258
- Anticipated Plasma Volume for Male = ((23.7 x height) + (9 x weight)) - 1709 ± 716
- Anticipated Plasma Volume for Female = ((40.5 x height) + (8.4 x weight)) - 4811 ± 392

$$RCM = Vol\ injected\ x\ \frac{(net\ STD\ wb\ x\ DF) - (net\ STD\ plasma\ x\ STD\ pct)}{(net\ wb) - (net\ plasma\ x\ (pt\ Pct))}\ x\ pt\ HCT$$

  - *Vol injected = volume injectd = 5 ml*
  - DF (Dilution Factor) = 50
  - Net counts = mean counts in cpm - background
  - Net STD whole blood = mean counts whole blood in cpm - background
  - Net STD plasma = mean counts standard plasma in cpm - background
  - STD Pct = standard plasmacrit in decimal = 1 - standard HCT
  - Pt Pct = patient plasmacrit = 1 - patient HCT

- Total Blood Volume (TBV) = RCM / (0.9xHCT)
- Plasma Volume = TBV - RCM
- Finding expressed as: ml/kg body weight

PV is measured using I-125-HAS (Human Serum albumin).

- Add 7 ml saline to 3 ml I-125 HSA
- Inject 5 ml I-125 HSA
- 5 ml blood is withdrawn into a heparinized syringe at 10, 20 and 30 minutes
- Centrifuge for 10 minute, 2500 RPM.
- Pipette 1 ml from plasma (10, 20 and 30 minutes) samples in to polystyrene tubes.
- Prepare plasma standard by adding 1 ml I-125 HAS to 99 ml water in a measurement cylinder.
- Pipette 1 ml from the standard in to polystyrene tubes.
- Prepare 6 polystyrene tubes:
  - Tube 1: pipette 1 ml water (for background)
  - Tube 2: 1 ml from the standard 100 ml measurement cylinder.
  - Tube 3: 1 ml from the standard 100 ml measurement cylinder.
  - Tube 4: 1 ml 10-minute plasma sample.
  - Tube 5: 1 ml 20-minute plasma sample.
  - Tube 6: 1 ml 30-minute plasma sample.
- Count the 6 tubes in a well counter
- spectrometer center 35 KeV.
- photo peak of I125.
- Count Time 300 seconds

Calculation:

- Plasma Volume = (5 x (DF x net STD plasma)) / net plasma samples

  - DF (Dilution Factor) = 100
  - net plasma samples = plasma samples at 10,20,30 minutes counts in cpm - background
  - Net STD plasma = standard plasma counts in cpm - background

10 Red Blood Cells Survival and Splenic Sequestration Rate Studies

Red Blood Cells Survival Study

- To measure red cells survival, a group of RBCs is followed by labeling (Cr-51 RBC labeling) to determine the elimination time from the circulation.
- This study can be done with Red Cell Mass (RCM) and Plasma Volume (PV) Measurements.

Indication

- Red blood cell survival:
    - Evaluation of lifespan of red blood cells
    - Effect of therapy on patients with hemolytic anemia.
- Splenic sequestration:
    - Evaluation of spleen in deceased red cell survival.

Procedure

Day 0:

- 10 ml blood with anticoagulant is drown from the patient for background.
- Add Cr-51 (150 µCi) (1.5 µCi/kg) to the blood.
- Incubate it for 20 min.
    - Add 50 mg ascorbic acid into the blood and incubate for 10 minutes. OR

- o   Centrifuge for 5 minute, 2500 RPM. Then remove the supernatant & add the same amount of saline & mix.
- Draw patient dose and inject to the patient.

After 24 hours:

A. Draw blood sample from the patient.
B. Check hematocrit for the sample.
C. Mark the heart, liver and spleen with indelible ink and acquire 10 minute counts over the marked areas with a counting probe.

- Repeat steps (A, B & C), on (2nd, 3rd, 5th, 7th, 10th, 13th, 15th, and 17th day)

Counting:

- After all the samples are collected:
- Prepare 10 polystyrene tubes:
  - o   Tube 1: pipette 1 ml patient background (Day 0)
  - o   Tube 2: 1 ml from Day 1 whole blood sample.
  - o   Tube 3: 1 ml from Day 2 whole blood sample.
  - o   Tube 4: 1 ml from Day 3 whole blood sample.
  - o   Tube 5: 1 ml from Day 5 whole blood sample.
  - o   Tube 6: 1 ml from Day 7 whole blood sample.
  - o   Tube 7: 1 ml from Day 10 whole blood sample.
  - o   Tube 8: 1 ml from Day 13 whole blood sample.
  - o   Tube 9: 1 ml from Day 15 whole blood sample.
  - o   Tube 10: 1 ml from Day 17 whole blood sample
- Count the 10 tubes in a well counter for 10 minutes
- spectrometer center 280-360 KeV.
- photo peak of Cr-51.

Calculation:

- $\% \, RBC \, Survival = \dfrac{\dfrac{net\ counts\ for\ that\ day}{Hct}}{net\ counts\ for\ the\ standard\ (day\ 1)} x100$
- Plot the samples counts on a graph.
- Divide day 0 counts by 2, then draw a horizontal line from until it intersect with the graph.
- Drop a vertical line from the intersection point, (it represent the time value for the mean survival rate of the RBCs.

- Normal values: 25-35 days.

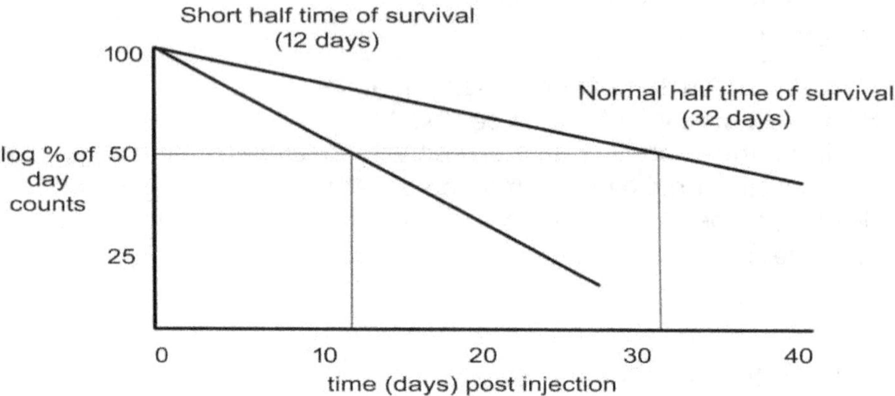

The samples count graph

Splenic Sequestration Rate Study

- Use the counting probe readings on heart, liver and spleen to calculate Splenic Sequestration Rate.
- Tc-99m SC images can also be obtained to locate the liver and spleen before obtaining Cr-51 surface counts.
- Use the following formula to calculate the radioactivity amount at any time in an organ:

$$Organ\ net\ activity =$$
$$organ\ counts\ at\ time\ t\ - \left(organ\ counts\ at\ time\ 0\ x\ \frac{Ht}{H0} \right)$$

Spleen to liver ratio = net spleen counts / net liver counts

Normal values: Spleen: liver ratio of 1:1, Spleen: Heart ratio of 1:1

11 Platelet Survival and Splenic Platelet Sequestration

Studies

Platelet survival Indications:

- investigate the mechanism of thrombocytopenia
- assess the effects of diseases and therapies on platelet survival
- Transplant rejection
- Image lesions with abnormal platelet uptake.
- Predict the success of splenectomy in AITP patients.

Platelet cell sequestration Indications:

- Determine if the splenic sequestration is the reason for reduced platelet number.

Radiopharmaceuticals:

- In-111-oxine
- Tc-99m HMPAO

Procedure:

- The labeling should be done in a sterile condition (inside Laminar air flow)
- 30-40 ml blood is drowning from the patient if the platelet count is normal.

- 100 ml blood is drawn from the patient if the platelet count is abnormal.
- Draw the blood in a syringe that contain ACD-A
- Mix the blood by turning the syringe end over.
- Centrifuge to remove RBC & WBC.
- Centrifuge to concentrate platelets by removing plasma & add the same amount of saline.
- Add 300-500 μCi In-111-oxine
- Centrifuge to removing unbound radionuclide (supernatant) & add the same amount of ACD saline.
- Reinject to the patient.
- QC 1: Calculate Labeling Efficiency.
- QC 2: Visual inspect for clots and clumps.
- QC 3: Radio labelling viability
  A. Heart & liver imaging
  B. Platelet Recovery should be 55-72% of the injected dose
- Collect 5 ml blood @ 60-minute post injection
- Calculate Recovery:

Platelet Recovery= ((blood concentration x blood volume x100) / injected dose

- obtaining samples at 20 min, 2 h, 3 h, and 4 h after injection and thereafter daily for up to 10 days.
- Counting of radioactivity using a well-type scintillator counter.
- calculate platelet survival.

Platelet cell sequestration study

- images are obtained over the liver and spleen.
- Anterior and posterior static images of the upper abdomen including the heart are obtained at 2, 48, 72, and 96 h after injection.
- SPECT images can also be obtained.

References

Part 1

- Technetium-99m Pharmaceuticals Preparation and Quality Control in Nuclear Medicine, Ilse Zolle, Springer
- The Radio Pharmacy a Technologist's Guide, European Association of Nuclear Medicine, 2008.
- Radiopharmacy: an update a technologist's guide, European Association of Nuclear Medicine.
- Nuclear medicine physics: the basics/Ramesh Chandra. -6th ed.
- Practical mathematics in nuclear medicine technology I Patricia Wells-2nd edition, Society of Nuclear Medicine.
- Package insert for DMSA, CURIUM.
- Package insert for MAG3, CURIUM.
- Package insert for HDP, CURIUM.
- Package insert for DTPA, CURIUM.
- Package insert for MIBI, CURIUM.
- Package insert for TIN COLLOID, CURIUM.
- Package insert for MAA, CURIUM.
- Package insert for NANO COLLOID, ROTOP.
- Package insert for BRIDA, POLATIC.

Part 2

- In-Vitro Studies, Nuclear Hematology, Lectures by Hind AL-Otaibi, Faculty of Allied Health, Kuwait University, 2019.
- IAEA, NUCLEAR HAEMATOLOGY, Chapter 26, by Johan S. Masjhur
- https://inis.iaea.org/collection/NCLCollectionStore/_Public/29/049/290 49621.pdf
- Nuclear Medicine Technology: Procedures and Quick References, Second Edition, Pete Shacktt.
- Nuclear Medicine Companion, Abdelhamid H. Elgazzar Ismet Sarikaya

OTHER AUTHOR PUBLICATIONS

- Nuclear Medicine Clinical Procedures for Technologists.

- CT in Nuclear Medicine.

Appendix A: Equations and Examples

- Equation for calculating the activity using the half-life:

$$A_t = A_0 e^{\dfrac{-0.693xt}{t\frac{1}{2}}}$$

  - A_t: Activity at specific time
  - A_0: Activity at time zero (original activity)
  - t: elapsed time
  - t1/2: half-life of the radioisotope
  - $\lambda = \dfrac{0.693}{t\frac{1}{2}}$

- Equation for calculating specific concentration:

$$\text{specific concentration} = \frac{\text{activity}}{\text{volume}}$$

- Equation for calculating volume required to have a needed activity:

$$\text{required volume ml} = \frac{\text{activity needed mCi}}{\text{specific concentration mCi/ml}}$$

- Calculating the volume of activity to be added to a kit:

  - Find the Tc 99m specific concentration
  - Find the kit required volume
  - Check if the calculated volume within the minimum and maximum accepted range for the kit
  - If the volume less than the minimum, then dilute the elute

- Calculating pediatric dose:

  - Clark's formula:

$$\text{Patient Dose} = \frac{\text{Patient Weight kg x Adult Dose}}{70 \text{ kg}}$$

- Calculating the patient dose:

  - Find the patient dose
  - Check if the calculated dose within the minimum and maximum accepted range
  - If the dose less than the minimum accepted dose, then use minimum dose.
  - If the dose more than the maximum accepted dose, then use maximum dose.

- **Example 1**
  A Tc99m elute with activity of 500 mCi, find the activity after 2 hours, given Tc99m t1/2= 6.01 hours?

$$A_t = A_o e^{\dfrac{-0.693 \times t}{t\frac{1}{2}}}$$

$$A_{2\ hour} = 500 e^{\dfrac{-0.693 \times 2}{6.01}} = 396.89 \text{ mCi}$$

- **Example 2**
  A 20 mCi Tc99m-Tetrofosmin patient dose needed after 2 hours, but must draw now, find the activity to be drawn now, given Tc99m t1/2= 6.01 hours?

$$A_t = A_o e^{\dfrac{-0.693 \times t}{t\frac{1}{2}}}$$

$$20 \text{ mCi} = A_o e^{\dfrac{-0.693 \times 2}{6.01}}, \qquad A_o = 20/0.79 = 25.31 mCi$$

- **Example 3**
  A Tc99m elute contains 600 mCi, in 11 ml, find the concentration?

$$\text{specific concentration} = \frac{\text{activity}}{\text{volume}}$$

  Tc99m elute concentration = 600/11= 54.54 mCi/ml

- **Example 4**
  Using example 3, if 100 mCi needed, find the volume to be drown?

$$\text{required volume ml} = \frac{\text{activity needed mCi}}{\text{specific concentration mCi/ml}}$$

volume = 100/54.54= 1.83ml

- **Example 5**
  If a Tc99m-Nano colloid kit need to be prepared with 35 mCi of elute. Find the volume to be added to the vial. Given the elute has 300 mci in 4ml. and minimum volume in the kit is 1ml?
    - Tc 99m specific concentration =300/4=75mCi/ml
    - The required volume = 35/75=.46ml
    - 0.46ml less than minimum volume in the kit,
    - 1ml-0.46ml=.54ml, so we draw 0.46ml elute and 0.54ml saline

- **Example 6**
  Find Tc99m-HDP patient dose and volume for a 50kg patient. the adult dose is 20mCi, kit concentration 25mCi/ml?

$$\text{Patient Dose} = \frac{\text{Patient Weight kg x Adult Dose}}{70 \text{ kg}}$$

Patient dose= (50x20)/70=14.28 mCi
Dose volume = 14.28/25= 0.57ml

Appendix B: Practical Work Sheet

- Elute 99Mo/99m Tc generator & calculate The elution concentration?
- Do the elution quality control?
    - QC 1: Radio Nuclide Purity (99Mo Break Through (ASSAY))
    - QC 2: Chemical Purity (ALUMINA Break Through)
    - QC 3: Radio Chemical Purity
- Prepare HIDA for two patients, 1st patient will be injected @ 10:30 am, 2nd patient will be injected @ 12:00 am, Now the time is 9:00am, and do QC?

Answer

Generator Elution:

We Need: saline vial, empty 11ml vial for Tc^{99m} & lead shield, forceps, alcohol wipe.

- Wipe the saline vial, then insert on its [lace on the generator
- Wipe 11ml vial, insert it inside lead shield, then insert it on the generator.
- After 2-3 min or after the bubbles on the saline vial stops, remove Tc^{99m} vial and recap the generator needle.
- Insert Tc^{99m} vial in the dose calibrator, measure activity, print label return vial in the lead shield & stick the label on it.
    - Elution Concentration:
    - E.X: 38.8 mCi in 10 ml @ 9:00 am

$$\text{specific concentration} = \frac{\text{activity}}{\text{volume}}$$

  - *=38.8/10= 3.8 mCi in 1 ml @ 9:00 am*

Elution Quality Control:

QC 1: Radio Nuclide Purity (99Mo Break Through (ASSAY)):

- Insert Empty lead on Dose calibrator & measure.
- Insert Tc^{99m} vial in lead, then Insert on Dose calibrator& measure.
- Insert Empty plastic dipper on Dose calibrator & measure.

- Insert Tc^{99m} vial in plastic dipper, then Insert on Dose calibrator& measure.

$$\frac{99Mo\ Activity\ \mu Ci}{99m\ Tc\ mCi} < 0.15\ \mu Ci\ per\ 1\ mCi\ of\ 99mTc\ \ should\ be\ between$$
$$< 0.01 - 0.015\ \mu Ci$$

- For QC2 & QC3: Draw 0.03ml of Elution in Insulin Syringe.

QC 2: Chemical Purity (<u>ALUMINA</u> Break Through):

- *From* <u>ALUMINA</u> Break Through QC kit, Take one strip
- Add a drop of standard AL^3 on the strip
- Add a drop of Tc^{99m} elution on the strip
  - AL^3 should be < 10 $\mu g\ in\ 1ml\ of$ Tc^{99m}

QC 3: Radio Chemical Purity:

Impurities Are: (Free Tc^{99m}, Hydrolyzed Tc02, Tc labelled to other compounds)

- Add 0.1ml of Acetone on a vial
- Add a drop of Tc^{99m} elution on a RED strip bottom line
- Put the strip on the Acetone Vial
- Wait until it moves to the top line
- Cut the strip on the middle line & put the two strips on two tubes & measure them.

Background	0.8 μCi	
Top free TCO4-	8.8μCi	8.8 - 0.8 = 8
Bottom TCO2-	1.2	1.2-0.8=0.4

$$\%\ Radiochemical\ Purity = \frac{Top}{Total} X100\ \ \ \ , should\ be\ between\ 90 - 95\%$$

=8/8.4*100=95.2 %

Prepare HIDA for two patients, 1st patient will be injected @ 10:30 am, 2nd patient will be injected @ 12:00 am, Now the time is 9:00am?

ANSWER:

- Take vial from the fridge, check Expiry Date
- Put it in shield and swap it.
- Calculate PT Dose:

- o Adult Dose for HIDA is (5 mCi)

$$A_t = A_o e^{\dfrac{-0.693 \times t}{t\frac{1}{2}}}$$

- o For 1st patient we should draw now
- o $5 = A_o e^{\frac{-0.693 \times 1.5}{6}}$, $A_O = 5.9 mCi$

- o For 2nd patient we should draw now

- o $5 = A_o e^{\frac{-0.693 \times 3}{6}}$, $A_O = 7 mCi$

- o 5.9 + 7 = 12.9 + 10% = 13 mCi, Min activity in HIDA kit is 10 mCi & Max activities is 40 mCi, so we add about 20 mci to HIDA vial.
- o Calculate Elution concentration NOW:
- o Elution Concentration is 3.8 mCi in 1 ml @ 9:00 am, NOW TIME is 9:30am
- o Volume of activity that we should add to HIDA vial @ 9:30am =

$$= \dfrac{20}{3.8 \times e^{\frac{-0.693 \times 3}{6}}} = 5.57 \text{ ml}$$

- Draw 5.57 ml from elution & add to HIDA vial, draw same amount of air, discard the syringe.
- Print label
- Shake and incubate for about 30 min

Qc for HIDA:

- Draw 0.03ml from Tc ^{99m} HIDA vial in Insulin Syringe.
- Add 0.1ml of H2o on a vial
- Add a drop on a blue strip bottom line
- Put the strip on the H2o Vial
- Wait until it moves to the top line
- Cut the strip on the middle line & put the two strips on two tubes & measure them.

- % Radiochemical IMPurity A $= \dfrac{\text{Top}}{\text{Total}} X100$

- Add 0.1ml of 20%Nacl on a vial
- Add a drop on an orange strip bottom line
- Put the strip on the 20%Nacl Vial
    - Wait until it moves to the top line
    - Cut the strip on the middle line & put the two strips on two tubes & measure them.

- % Radiochemical IMPurity $B = \dfrac{\text{Top}}{\text{Total}} X100$

- % Radiochemical Purity $= 100 - (A + B)$ should $> 90\%$

- Draw Dose for the two patients:
- Tc ^{99m} HIDA activity 18.3 mCi in 5.6 ml @ 9:30 am, NOW TIME is 9:42am
- Tc ^{99m} HIDA concentration = 18.3/5.6=3.2679 3.26 mCi/ml

- For first patient we should draw now

$$A = \frac{5.9}{3.26 \times e^{\frac{-0.693 \times 12 \text{ min}}{360 \text{ min}}}} = 1.8 \text{ ml}$$

- For 2nd patient we should draw now

$$A = \frac{7}{3.26 \times e^{\frac{-0.693 \times 15 \text{ min}}{360 \text{ min}}}} = 2.2 \text{ ml}$$

- Draw the dose for the two patient, & put it in a shield

Appendix C: EANM Guidelines on Radio pharmacy radiation protection and good practice methods[1]

Some points related to Radio pharmacy radiation protection and good practice methods:

- Only licensed personnel are authorized to handle and use radiopharmaceuticals.
- The general principles of radiation protection are:
    - Justification: All procedures involving radioactive material must be justified.
    - Optimization: The radiation exposure to any individual should be as low as reasonably achievable, ALARA principle.
    - Limitation: The radiation dose received by the personnel handling radioactive material will never exceed the legally established dose limits.
- The basic principles for reduction of radiation doses:
    - Time: The shorter the time of exposure to radiation, the lower the dose to the operator.
    - Distance: The radiation dose decreases with a factor equal to the square root of the distance from the radiation source. The operator's distance from the source can be increased by using forceps, tongs, or manipulators in handling the radioactive material.
    - Shielding: The radiation dose can be reduced by placing shielding material between the source and the operator. For protection against gamma radiation, walls made of heavy concrete or lead

---

[1] The Radio Pharmacy a Technologist's Guide, European Association of Nuclear Medicine, 2008.
Radiopharmacy: an update a technologist's guide, European Association of Nuclear Medicine.

bricks are used. For transport containers material such as tungsten may be used for higher energy gamma irradiation radionuclides, giving a higher shielding per weight unit when compared to lead.

- Work practices in the radio pharmacy should be standardized and The procedures should be documented and made readily available to those working in the radio pharmacy.
- Good pharmaceutical practice should be applied in radiopharmaceuticals preparation.
  - All manipulation of radioactive materials should be done, using aseptic techniques, within the shielded contained workstation or laminar flow cabinet.
  - In an area where unsealed radioactive substances are used, no food or drink, cosmetic or smoking materials, crockery or cutlery should be brought.
- All staff classified as radiation workers must wear a personal dosimeter (TLD, film badge, electronic dosimeter).
- A finger TLD to monitor extremity dose should be used by staff preparing and handling radioactive materials.
- Before handling radioactive substances:
  - staff should ensure that they wash their hands,
  - any cut or break in the skin should be covered.
  - Protective coats or gowns should be worn.
  - Disposable gowns offer benefits in terms of maintaining sterility.
  - Gloves must always be removed and disposed of as radioactive waste after handling radioactive materials.
  - After removal of gloves, Hands should be washed again.
  - Upon leaving the radio pharmacy, disposable gowns should be removed and stored as radioactive waste until monitoring confirms that they are at background radiation levels.
- To reduce staff dose, protective equipment, when handling radioactive materials, should be used.
- Equipment for increase the distance from the source:
  - tongs and forceps
  - syringe shields
  - vial shields
  - drip trays to decrease spillage contamination
  - shielded syringe carriers
  - decontamination kit

- The equipment should be stored outside the laminar flow cabinet and should be cleaned regularly.
- All of the materials required should be assembled and placed in or close to the contained workstation/LAFC, before starting the preparation and dispensing of radiopharmaceuticals.
- All vials containing radioactive materials must be shielded while handling.
- vials should only be removed from their shields for assay, inspection or disposal.
- All syringes containing radioactive liquids must be shielded while handling, except during an assay.
- Long handled tongs should be used to handle unshielded vials or syringes.
- If a spill occurs, then it should be cleaned up before proceeding any further.
- All items that might be contaminated should be removed from the affected area and stored safely.
- If the contaminated items are not required immediately, allow natural decay to take care of the contamination.
- If the items are needed, they should be cleaned with alcohol swabs.
- The manufacturer's recommendations should be followed for reconstitution of pharmaceutical kits.
- Kits Protective caps should be removed and the vials should be placed in a labeled vial shields.
- The rubber septum of the vial should be swabbed with alcohol.
- To reconstitute the pharmaceutical a shielded (5 or 10 ml) syringes capped with 21G needles should be used.
- The appropriate activity and volume of 99mTc solution should be added to each vial.
- The pharmaceutical should be allowed to incubate for the specified length of time.
- When adding 99mTc solution or saline to a vial, equivalent volume of air should be withdrawn to equalize the pressure.
- The activity and volume of 99mTc solution added to each pharmaceutical should be recorded.
- patient injections should be withdrawn using shielded 2ml syringes capped with 21G.
- The patient activity must be within 10% of the required activity.
- Patient injections should be in a volume of 1ml.

- If the volume is below 1m, Saline may be used to increase the volume.
- Some injections volume can be less or more than 1ml, in this case the manufacturer's instructions should be followed.
- When the patient injection is prepared, the air in the syringe must be expelled while the needle is capped.
- If there is a droplet of liquid visible in the needle cap, replace the needle and cap.
- Each patient injection must be measured, recorded and labeled with an appropriate label (patient name, scan type, activity to be administered, date and time of injection).

Appendix D: EANM Guidelines on Waste management procedures[2]

Waste management procedures points:

- Non-radioactive waste should be separated from radioactive waste and disposed of as normal hospital waste.
- Shielded waste bins should be lined with plastic liners that can be easily removed.
- Technetium 99m waste: the duration of storage will be determined by its half-life of 6.02 hours.
- Longer lived waste should be stored separately.
- Radioactive waste generated daily: includes syringes, elution vials, pharmaceutical vials, needles and swabs.
- Waste arising from the preparation and dispensing of radiopharmaceuticals should be primarily disposed in the waste bin built into the contained workstation/LAFC.
- Some bulky items such as paper waste and gloves with no risk of contamination may be disposed in a shielded waste bin outside the cabinet.
- Radioactive waste contaminated by blood should be removed to a shielded bin outside the cabinet.
- The waste container in the workstation should be emptied before starting work in the cabinet, when the waste in the bin has decayed overnight.
- Segregation of waste according to half-life is good practice.

---

[2] The Radio Pharmacy a Technologist's Guide, European Association of Nuclear Medicine, 2008.
Radiopharmacy: an update a technologist's guide, European Association of Nuclear Medicine.

- Paper waste Any gloves used in the cabinet or used to handle blood or isotopes will be considered to be contaminated.
- Paper tray liners in the cabinet or paper used to clean surfaces in the cabinet are also considered to be contaminated.
- Contaminated gloves and paper should be disposed in a shielded bin if there is no biological contamination (blood or plasma).
- If there is a biological contamination, the waste should be placed in a sharps bin, using tongs.
- For long term storage of waste, the waste should be removed from the shielded bin, labeled with details of the contents and stored as radioactive waste in a designated store.
- Sharps bins Syringes, needles, butterflies etc. should be disposed of after use to shielded sharps bins.
- Full sharps bins should be closed, marked 'radioactive', dated and removed to the radioactive waste store.
- Disposal of waste All radioactive waste - sharps bins, paper waste, ventilation kits - should be securely stored and monitored regularly.
- Waste should be checked by using a suitable meter in a low background environment and should be disposed of, once it has decayed to background level.
- Any items above background should be retained for a further period of decay in storage.
- All radioactive warning labels should be removed from waste, prior to disposal in hospital waste.

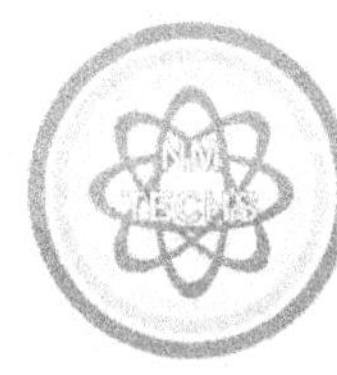

NM Techs™

Educational Recourses for Nuclear Medicine Technologists

Telegram: NM_Techs
YouTube: NM_Techs
Twitter: Nm_Techs
Instagram: nm_techs
Facebook: NM Techs
Threads: nm_techs
Email: nm.techs.kh@gmail.com

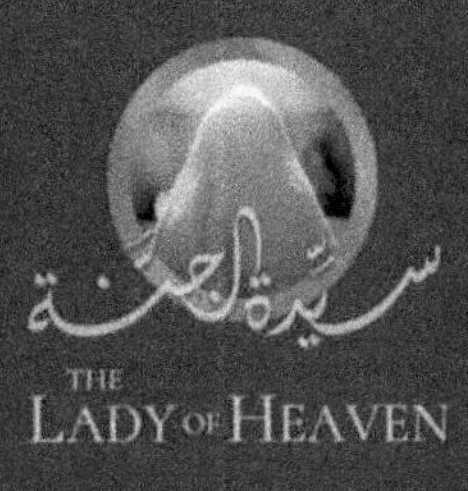

ماذا على من شمّ تربة أحمد   أن لا يشمّ مدى الزّمان غواليا
صبّت عليّ مصائب لو أنّها   صبّت على الأيّام صرن لياليا
قل للمغيّب تحت أطباق الثّرى   إن كنت تسمع صرختي وندائيا
قد كنت ذات حمى بظلّ محمّد   لا أخش من ضيم وكان جماليا
فاليوم أخضع للذّليل واتّقي   ضيمي وأدفع ظالمي بردائيا
فاذا بكت قمريّة في ليلها   شجنا على غصن بكيت صباحيا
فلأجعلنّ الحزن بعدك مونسي   ولأجعلنّ الدّمع فيك وشاحيا

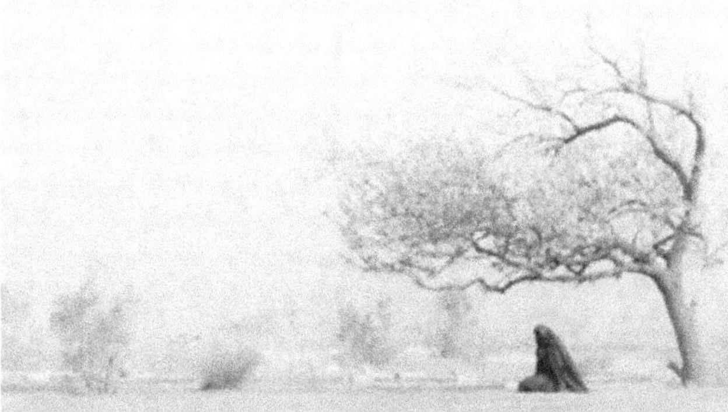